Contents

Birth of a Book 1

11th Commandment 5

Spiritual Autobiography 8

I Wasn't There, or Was I? 11

Did I Get the Wrong Channel? 15

Searching for Something.. 18

Have We Lived Before? 22

Flying with the Eagles 27

Coming Home to Myself 32

Without Even a GPS 36

The Search aka Chronology of the Disease 43

Illusion of Invulnerability 49

I Guess They Didn't Like the Food 52

Fired Without Cause 58

Another Brush with Death 62

Invisibility 65

Why Can't I Stand? 71

Living Alone Has Its Hazards 74

Setting Your Intentions 81

Drama of the Day aka Life in a Bubble 88

Physically Challenged? 95

God Doesn't Give You More Than You Can Handle 100

Another Commandment Broken 103

Dark Night of the Soul 108
No Call, No Show Is No Good 112
Expect the Unexpected 115
Equipment Failure 121
Pilot Error or Mechanical Failure 128
You Need to Get Away 133
Taking the Simple Things for Granted 138
The High Cost of Reality 144
Tongue-In-Cheek 150
What is the Lesson? 153
Why Did I Choose Judaism? 156
What is in a Name? 160
Prayer for Healing 163
Tribute to Debbie Friedman 165
About the Author 166

Acknowledgments

I have backed away from writing this book each time I have started it. It is intensely personal. It is self-revealing. It is difficult for me to be this vulnerable, this open, but I know it's time that the book is written. It would be easier to write fiction than nonfiction that is so intensely personal, but I feel driven to do it.

I've heard an elephant is pregnant for two years. The writing of this book has been a twenty-year pregnancy! Way too long to have an elephant in the room. It's about time the elephant emerges from the womb.

Many thanks to my partner, Kirie, for her encouragement, love, and support. She is my rock. Whenever I feel down, she lifts me up. I also appreciate the love and support from my friend and Rabbi, Alicia Magal. She is my spiritual mentor.

My mother has been instrumental in providing emotional support and encouragement throughout my entire life and has always believed in me. My father provided well for the family and made sure I received a college education.

Many thanks to Alison Twist Yarger for the long hours of editing and correction – you helped me tremendously. Our high school English teacher would be proud! My psychic friend, Cynthia Hart-Button, provided artwork for the covers and pushed my buttons until I got this done. I am grateful for her nagging. Anita Rosenfield spent hours carefully editing my draft and making awesome suggestions. I appreciate her skills and expertise. Her friendship and encouragement provided enthusiasm for the final editing push. Additionally, I want to thank my friends and family who have supported and loved me throughout this journey we call life.

When you have spent the majority of your adult life using a chair for mobility, you see life from a different perspective. *View from a Chair* is being written to share my personal experiences of disability, of caregivers, of despair, and of hope. By no means do I believe I have all of the answers. All I have are life experiences dealing with my disability and the problems associated with it. Hopefully this book will help others in a similar situation.

© Copyright 2018 by Marilyn Gard

All Rights Reserved

Birth of a Book

I woke up this morning after an absolutely fantastic dream. I was at a women's conference, and unbeknownst to me, I was one of the speakers. I went to the conference room where I was supposed to speak and sat in the back of the room wondering "what the hell am I doing here?" Then I looked at the flyer and realized I was supposed to be speaking on conflict resolution.

"Great," I thought.

"Whip up a seminar in the next five minutes. No problem, I can do it." I shook my head in bewilderment.

"How did I forget I was supposed to speak today?"

I looked down at my clothes. I was wearing my favorite flannel shirt from forty years ago. Brown plaid, somewhat faded because I'd worn it so often. I guess that happens to everything that's your favorite, whether it be clothes, a book, a keepsake. They look faded and worn over time. But you don't necessarily want to replace them. Our society has become so used to everything being expendable, replaceable. Not my flannel shirt!

"Oh well," I thought.

I didn't have to time to change clothes.

"The show must go on."

As I sat in the back of the room, I formatted the seminar. I knew I wanted it to be participatory because I certainly didn't have time to prepare a lecture in the next five minutes. As I looked around, I saw there were only 6 or 8 people in the room.

"At least it isn't intimidating," my mind reasoned. "I should be able to wing it for this small crowd."

I prepared different scenarios in my head, much like the TV show *What Would You Do?* If you were in a situation where you need to have a voice, an opinion, or intervene in an untenable situation, what would you do? If you saw someone disparaged or publicly humiliated, what would you do?

So, as I sat at the back of the room, I came up with situations in my head. For example, if you were a supervisor and saw two employees arguing vehemently about something, what would you do? You couldn't hear the argument because you were far enough away you couldn't distinguish the words. And besides that, you were somewhat hard of hearing so that made it more difficult. How would you handle that situation so it didn't affect the entire workplace? How would you resolve the conflict?

I then thought of another scenario. You were the supervisor and you knew an employee was stealing from the company. You were pretty sure you know which employee it was - but you had no direct evidence. How would you handle that situation?

I looked down at myself sitting in the chair realizing that once again I had to conduct a seminar from a chair. At this time, more and more people were filing into the room to the point where nearly every chair was filled. By the time I looked up, 30 or 40 people must have entered the room.

"Great." One part of my brain was amused, the other half was frightened.

I was going to conduct a seminar I was totally unprepared for, dressed inappropriately as a workshop leader for a room filling with people. Besides, I had to throw my voice over the crowd to make myself heard because I had no microphone. I hadn't led a seminar in years. This was going to be fun! Not...

As my mind alternated between various conflicts I could throw out to the room for discussion, and the panic I felt because I wasn't prepared, I thought again about my situation.

"What would you do if your life suddenly changed and you were forced to be in a wheelchair for the rest of your life? How would you handle it?" Obviously, the biggest conflicts we will ever face in our lives are the ones that are internal and personal. In the final scenario of our session that day, I was going to describe different scenarios coming from my own personal life of being in a chair.

"That's not appropriate," my mind interjected. "Don't make it about you."

"Why not?" another voice interceded.

"Why not a make it about real life? It's true you can never really walk in someone else's moccasins but go ahead and give people a short window through which to view your life. At some point as they age, they may have to face it as well."

At that point, I woke from my dream and was absolutely amazed at its complexity and clarity. That's why I had to write about it in this book. In fact, that's the reason I'm writing this book – in case you ever find yourself with a chronic health problem and have to decide how to respond to it.

I have started this book many times over the past twenty years. I started to write in earnest a year ago. My dream told me one thing crystal clear: stop procrastinating and get it done! No more lame excuses.

11th Commandment

During Shabbat services one Friday night, the Rabbi was talking about the Ten Commandments or Ten Utterances elucidated in Exodus. As she stated, we all know we need to live by the Ten Commandments; that is a given for most of us. It doesn't matter what your religious beliefs are - or even if you have any. The Ten Commandments provide a guide to an honorable way of life regardless of your spirituality.

After reading from the Torah, the rabbi suggested that we each have an 11th commandment known only to us. It might be to work at the food bank, help abused women, volunteer at the Humane Society or any other worthy cause. We would each know intuitively what our 11th commandment is because it is unique to each individual. As soon as she said that, the song by Debbie Friedman echoed in my head. As with so many of her songs, this particular song tells a Torah story through music; it puts to music the direction that God gave to Abraham and Sarah.

L'chi lach, to a land that I will show you
Leich l'cha, to a place you do not know
L'chi lach, on your journey I will bless you

And (you shall be a blessing) l'chi lach
And (you shall be a blessing) l'chi lach
And (you shall be a blessing) l'chi lach

L'chi lach, and I shall make your name great
Leich l'cha, and all shall praise your name

L'chi lach, to the place that I will show you
(L'sim-chat cha-yim) l'chi lach
(L'sim-chat cha-yim) l'chi lach
(L'sim-chat cha-yim) l'chi lach

I immediately knew my 11th commandment: **make your life a blessing.** As soon as I realized the impact of the commandment, I started to bargain with God. I'm obviously not nearly as spiritually elevated as Abraham or Sarah.

"Make my life a blessing? Can you be a little more specific, God?" If my mission is to feed the hungry, I know how to bring food to the synagogue to go to the food pantry. If my mission is to help neglected animals, I have a clue how to do it and support the Humane Society or other rescue organizations. But make my life a blessing? How do I do that? I didn't hear a thunderous voice in response. I didn't see a burning bush to light the way.

Make my life a blessing? How do I do that? There is no guidebook. There's no manual I can read. I'm sure there's no video tutorial on YouTube.

It's my hope that reading this book will help someone, even one person, realize he or she is not alone when dealing with chronic illness or disability. *View from a Chair* is a book about my personal experiences living the majority of my adult life from the perspective of a wheelchair. It's part of my 11th commandment, to make my life a blessing. Lech Lacha – go on a journey to yourself. This book chronicles my journey.

My personal tribute to Debbie Friedman. I set her music to a slideshow of our beautiful synagogue and Rabbi: https://youtu.be/sAm6auDe3T0

Spiritual Autobiography

I grew up in a farm community thirteen miles from the closest town. Next door to my house was a small United Methodist Church. I was reared going to Sunday school and church services. Because I started playing piano when I was five, I started playing piano for Sunday school by the time I was 10. Soon, I was playing the organ for the church services.

As a teenager, I sought a personal relationship with God. In addition to the Sunday services, I went to Wednesday night prayer meeting. I was the only teenager interested in that much religiosity. I became president of the Youth Fellowship and of the Bible Club in my high school. At the age of 16, I was "saved," a born again Christian. For those who never grew up with a fundamentalist background, it is a process of responding to an altar call where you accept Jesus as your personal savior. A year later, I was "filled with the Holy Spirit" at a similar church service. Quite frankly, I never really knew what it meant to be filled with the Holy Spirit. It was just the next step of declaration of my Christianity.

At the age of seventeen, I went off to a fundamentalist Christian college. I wasn't really sure what I wanted to major in, but I had thoughts of becoming a minister or a missionary. Everything changed when I fell in love with the Dean of Women who was also my therapist, basketball coach, and professor. Yes, I was sexually naïve at seventeen. It took me totally by surprise.

The new-found love of my life couldn't handle the Christian guilt of being a lesbian. She told other professors and eventually the Dean of Men. One night while I was in the laundry room of the dorm, the Dean of Men came in and confronted me. I was alone. No one else was doing laundry at the time.

"My wife and I were very much in love when we were dating but we waited until marriage to consummate our love," he said.

"We didn't want to hold out for marriage to have sex, but we did."

Then he confronted me with the words that stung my soul for years to come. "Homosexuality is an abomination against God."

Obviously, he'd heard about my relationship with the Dean of Women. "You will surely go to hell if you continue this behavior."

I turned every shade of red as the shame and humiliation and guilt infiltrated every cell of my body. I shattered like glass; my soul was fractured.

""Promise you won't do 'it' again," the Dean of Men admonished me.

"I won't," I promised, not knowing what "it" was.

At that point in time, I didn't know he had paraphrased the passage in Leviticus to do the most psychological damage to me. This phrase, taken out of historical context and mistranslated, continues to be used as a self-righteous sword against the LGBT community by many people professing Christianity.

I have one response to those individuals who have never truly studied that passage.

"Shame on you."

I later made it my personal mission to investigate the true meaning of the passage.

I Wasn't There, or Was I?

The humiliation started an intense period in my life where guilt and shame predominated. I was going to burn in hell for my sins. Because the object of my love could not handle the guilt, she got married between my freshman and sophomore years of college. Marriage was her attempt to go straight. I remember going to her two days before her wedding, begging her not to do it. This was in July. I have no memory of my sophomore year of college. In fact, I didn't even know I lost a year until we reconnected 10 years later.

We were sitting in the living room talking one day and I asked "Why didn't you invite me to the wedding?"

"What do you mean? You were there. You played piano while Audrey sang." She looked at me quizzically.

"No way." I shook my head vehemently.

"Why would I lie about something like that? I have a picture here, do you want to see it?"

I was confused and dumbfounded. "I wasn't there. Why are you making this up?" By this time, I was getting angry.

With that statement, she got up from the couch and started rummaging around in dresser drawers in the bedroom. Eventually, she came out of the bedroom with a wedding album in hand. I didn't believe her until I saw the picture. Yes, I attended the wedding. I recognized the dress. Still, it jogged no memory of the event as it was totally blocked from my mind. The brain it is extraordinary in the many ways it can protect us from a complete break by taking over in times of stress. I have the transcripts of my sophomore year of college but not a single memory of it. None. I went through one entire year in a dissociative state.

The amazing part of a dissociative state is the fact you seem to function perfectly fine on a day-to-day basis. I obviously attended classes. I have the grades to show for it. I obviously slept, ate, and went about a daily routine – but was totally disconnected from it.

I switched colleges at the end of my sophomore year and began a new period in my life where I questioned God. I felt abandoned by Christianity. I felt abandoned by God. I turned away from my faith, turning my back on both Christianity and God. I threw the baby out with the bathwater. I asked the question just about every lesbian or gay person asks "Why was I born this way?" It would be so much easier to be heterosexual. Quite frankly, I was angry at God.

For many years, questions swirled around me like a dust storm, blocking my view.

"Why had God made me this way? If I was in His/Her image, was He/She also gay?" Considering the rhetoric that permeates the political climate nowadays, wouldn't that be a kicker? Wouldn't it be a real slap in the face to learn God sees only love and not gender? That is my personal belief.

After being shamed and humiliated, I stayed away from church. I stayed away from Christians. I didn't want any part of the guilt and shame that had so dominated my entry into my sexual orientation. The only thing I held onto was the fact that what I experienced was love...how could that be wrong?

Looking back now, I would have to describe the next forty years of my life as wandering in the desert. I tried many things. I joined a women's spirituality group in which we explored pagan rituals. This was back in the '70s and early '80s during the hippie days. We met every week. When I turned 27, I started experiencing symptoms of multiple sclerosis. By the time I was in my mid-30s, I was chair bound.

I remember one particularly poignant meeting where one of the group members declared "I would rather be dead than disabled."

Then, realizing what she had said, she turned to me. "I'm so sorry."

My response was simple. "I don't think it's a matter of choice. You have to play the hand you're dealt."

I think that philosophy has been pivotal in helping me get through the challenges I have faced. I can't control the hand I was dealt; I can only control my reaction to it.

Did I Get the Wrong Channel?

During this time, I attended summer and winter solstice celebrations. During my mid-30s, I began to explore the metaphysical. I was invited to channeling sessions where a woman named Mary channeled Chief Joseph. Chief Joseph was the tribal chief of the Nez Perce tribe of northwestern Oregon. He became famous for leading his people in an epic flight across the Rocky Mountains after being ordered to relocate to a reservation.

After years of being chased and fighting, he spoke these now-famous words. "Hear me, my chiefs: My heart is sick and sad. From where the sun now stands, I will fight no more forever."

During the channeling session, everyone in the room had opportunities to ask a question. When my turn came, I asked the question foremost in my mind. "Why am I in the chair in this lifetime?"

I was still struggling to come to grips with it. I had been in the chair three or four years by that time.

"You chose this at the age of four."

"What? Why would I choose that?" I was incredulous. It seemed like an irresponsible and foolish choice. I couldn't believe my ears.

"I don't know. I can't tell you." Mary shook her head as the words of Chief Joseph flowed through her.

I was given no answer as to why. Why would I choose to be in the chair? I left the channeling session more confused than when I entered. If this had been a TV show, I would have switched channels!

As part of my spiritual search, I attended classes taught by Mary. She herself had gone through extensive training learning to channel. As part of the class, I explored channeling my spirit guide. His name was Ottumweah – I am not sure about the spelling. In a past life, Ottumweah was my husband and we had two sons. They were handsome boys with straight, polished onyx hair that fell halfway down their backs. Ottumweah was a medicine man in our tribe although I do not know which tribe that was. By Native American standards, he was a big guy. He would go to the streams and rivers to catch fish with his bare hands. During one meditation, I saw him break the ice in the stream so he could reach in and grab the fish. Maybe that is why Colorado always felt like home to me. I think we may have lived there at one point in time.

In 1874, we were attacked by another tribe. Ottumweah hid our sons and me behind bushes as he fought the attackers. I saw the whole fight. He died by a spear to the abdomen; he was killed in front of me. After he died, I took my two beautiful boys to another part of the country. We built a cabin in the meadow where I lived with them until they were grown. I was never with another man. After my sons got married and left my home, I was alone. I visualized this whole scene one day almost as if I was attending a movie.

To this day, Ottumweah is with me. One day during my regular biweekly visit, Dr. Jan, my chiropractor, saw him standing over my right shoulder. "Are you aware that often a man accompanies you to your visits?" she asked. "He is a large guy and looks like a medicine man."

"Yep, I know him intimately," I answered. I explained everything I had seen, our life together and his death. "What I don't understand is this – why is he not with me in this lifetime?"

"He said he is always with you in spirit."

I believe that. I often feel his presence. I sometimes wish he would have reincarnated with me in this lifetime. I guess there were lessons I needed to learn on my own.

Searching for Something

During this period of my life, I channeled Ottumweah frequently. Sometimes, I would channel for a group of people who would ask questions. Even though I was physically present during a channeling, the answers were sometimes startling. One of the amazing aspects of channeling is that you get to see pictures – it's like watching a movie where Ottumweah would describe the scenes to the person asking the question. After coming out of trance, I wouldn't remember the questions but I *would* remember the picture shows.

The most difficult thing for me was channeling for family and friends. If they asked questions, I wanted to make sure they weren't my answers. I wanted to make sure the answers came from spirit.

One night I channeled for my mother and her friend, Kathy. My mother asked Ottumweah about the birthmark on her leg. His response was immediate.

"During the Civil War, you were a soldier. During one of the battles, you were struck by a bayonet."

"Did I die?"

"No, you did not die from the wound but you did lie on the battlefield for two days before they could get to you."

Quite honestly, I couldn't have made this up. I didn't remember the birthmark on her leg, even where it was on the lower part of her leg. She has always been fascinated with the Civil War. She likes reading historical novels set during that time. Her attraction to Civil War history all made sense to me now.

Her friend Kathy was a former nun. She asked about one of the sisters who had died. They had lived together in the convent and worked together.

"I have often wondered how she is doing."

"She wants me to tell you everything is great. She is singing and dancing, almost like the *Sound of Music*."

"Does she feel good?"

"She's very happy. She wants you to know that she loves you."

After I came out of the trance, Kathy explained to me that this particular sister was a very loving soul. Later in life, she experienced crippling rheumatoid arthritis so extreme she could barely move. Despite her disability, she never complained. It was a source of great comfort to know she could now dance.

On one particularly eventful night, I channeled Ottumweah while Mary channeled Chief Joseph. A group of people gathered for the session. At one point, the two of them (Ottumweah and Chief Joseph) started talking back and forth, exchanging greetings and talking about their lives. Words I didn't understand and could barely pronounce were coming out of my mouth. As people watched and listened, the two spirits talked back and forth for five minutes in native tongue. Neither Mary nor I understood the words, but everyone in the room understood the content and the energy they exchanged. It was pure love.

For the next two days, I was left with the most incredible feeling of unconditional love I have ever experienced. Words cannot describe what happened that night. The energy they exchanged was phenomenal.

During this time, I also learned to pull energy from Mother Earth and leave my body during meditation. Because it is so pleasant to leave my body behind, I don't allow myself to do it often. Who wouldn't want to leave behind a body that has strange sensations and the inability to respond to the simplest commands? I also learned to pull up energy and use it to heal other people. I never have been able to use it to heal myself, it just seems Spirit says "No" when I try. So I have stopped trying.

While I really enjoyed channeling, my partner was jealous. Channeling requires the ability to let go, knowing you have set boundaries for any entity to use your body. You have to be willing to allow spirit come through and feel comfortable with that choice. Because of my partner's jealousy and her inability to successfully channel, I gave up channeling to maintain the relationship. I regret that choice. I have a tendency to give myself up in personal relationships; this was yet another instance my putting relationship above my own needs. Unfortunately, women experience this phenomenon too often, granting priority to the relationship over her individual needs.

I read about Zen Buddhism. I also studied Hopi spirituality and have since developed a good friend who lives on First Mesa. As an elder, she has explained their rituals and tribal dances. I built a medicine wheel in my backyard and retreat to pray since it helps to connect me with the universe. Whenever energy becomes heavy in my home, I burn sage and sweetgrass to clear the negative energy. Many of the Native rituals seem familiar and comfortable to me. On at least two occasions, I have experienced past lives where I have been Native American. My heartbeat resonates with drumming circles and chanting. With the beat of the drum, I am transported to another time, another place.

Have We Lived Before?

For years, the topic of past lives as been hotly discussed and debated. Have we really lived before? If we have, what were those lives like?

Sometimes when you meet someone for the first time, there seems to be an unexplainable familiarity, almost like déjà vu. You immediately feel comfortable. You don't experience awkward silences because you always have something to say to each other. Did you have a past life together? Maybe!

Through online dating, I met a woman who lives in Toronto. We experienced an immediate, unexplainable connection. After talking one night, I saw our past life together and began to understand the connection.

We lived on the second story of a flat. The doorway was at least ten feet tall with a ledge on the top. We were married; I was her husband. I was an accountant who didn't enjoy accounting but stuck with it anyway because I needed to support us. The streets were cobblestone, rough and bumpy. The neighborhood could best be described as shabby, a working class neighborhood. I rode an old-time bicycle back and forth to work.

One night, I saw myself riding back to our flat and securing the bicycle against the post in front of the building. I bounded up the stairs to the smell of cinnamon. When I entered our kitchen, I was greeted with the unmistakable smell of homemade cinnamon rolls. While planting a kiss on her, I tried to reach behind her to grab one of the rolls she had just pulled from the oven. She slapped my hand, and not very gently! I relished the fact that we were playful with each other. Because she was always baking, I teased her relentlessly about the flour that consistently decorated her apron.

I looked around the room. The kitchen, dining room and living room were all one big room. We had a secondhand couch against a large bay window in the front of the apartment. I saw her sketchpad lying on the table next to the couch. "Did you have fun drawing today?"

She nodded her head and smiled. "The light was just perfect. How marvelous to sit in the sun and draw the trees outside our window," she exclaimed.

I was privileged to watch a full length movie of our past life. I won't divulge all of the details. Suffice it to say, after we ate dinner, we retired to the bedroom. There is one detail that was particularly interesting though. Before lying on the bed, she forced me to take off the bedspread. I wasn't even allowed to sit on the bed until the bedspread was removed.

After seeing that past life, I sat at my computer and dictated the whole story. While sharing it with her the next day, she told me she always bakes with cinnamon... lots of different things. Cinnamon rolls, cinnamon strudel, apple pie, cinnamon cakes. Being brought up in Italy for the first few years of her life, she learned to bake with cinnamon since it is common for that portion of Italy. She also confirmed other details that I had seen in my vision.

"How did you know I will never lie on the bed without taking the bedspread off?" she asked. "That is just a quirk of mine. I never want shoes to be on the bed or even blue jeans."

"I didn't know that. I just saw it. It was part of the show."

In that lifetime, she died in her forties. She had a weak respiratory system and which was the cause of her death. I was distraught and lonely but I never married again. In this lifetime, she often gets colds and bronchitis in the winter. Of course, who wouldn't if they lived in Canada? I'm entitled to say that because I live in Arizona by choice after having grown up in Michigan.

A few days later she sent a picture of Strasbourg, France. When she visited there, she didn't want to leave southern France. She didn't know why. She just felt she had come home. After looking at the picture, I googled Strasbourg. I found a 50-scene slideshow of the city. On the second slide, I saw a picture of the street that could have been the exact location of our flat. The streets were cobblestone. On the left side of the picture, there was a flat with a tall door and overhanging ledge. The second story had a bay window. Truly, the only difference was the color of the building. What I saw in my vision was a blue building; the online version was gray. I wish I could have visited that street and that building and bounded up the stairs again. Would I have returned home? I think so.

This story is ironic because we still haven't met in this lifetime, but we keep in touch regularly and know without a doubt that we love each other. I know our friendship has endured throughout the years and was rekindled by a chance meeting on an online dating service.

Some people attempt to use hypnosis for past life regression. My one experience with hypnotic regression was unsuccessful. The hypnotist started by having me walk down a flight of stairs. That is a typical method of inducing hypnosis. For anyone who has instability or gait problems, walking down is much more difficult than walking up steps, a path, or any type of surface. While walking up is more strenuous physically, walking down requires more balance.

Most of my past life experiences have happened while channeling for other people or seeing spontaneous movies of my own past lives. Yes, I believe we have lived before and our soul will continue to live after the physical body wears out.

Flying with the Eagles

If you have never been to Sedona, Arizona, you owe it to yourself to be one of the three to four million tourists who visit here every year. I visited Sedona for the first time when I was in my middle 30's. After meeting my psychic friend, Cynthia, in Michigan, I decided to come for a visit. Cynthia lived in Sedona for many years prior to taking responsibility for the white buffalo herd and moving with them to find an appropriate permanent residence.

During my vacation, I went down to Red Rock Crossing, now called Crescent Moon Park. The cover of this book is a picture of Cathedral Rock which can be viewed and hiked from red Rock Crossing. The city of Sedona is known for vortex energy and Cathedral Rock happens to be one of the most powerful vortices in the area.

My friend Jackie accompanied me on this trip. "Would it be all right with you if I walked along the water for a while?" she asked.

As much as I wanted to, I knew I couldn't get close to the creek on any of the hiking trails with my power chair.

"Sure," I responded.   "I'll bask in the sun and enjoy the scenery."

As she disappeared from view, I pulled my wheelchair off to the side of the narrow sidewalk where I wouldn't be disturbed by other tourists. I decided to meditate, pulling energy from Mother Earth. I had learned to leave my body as part of channeling, so pulling up energy in the sacred space happened easily.

Before I realized what had happened, I was in the air alongside a beautiful eagle. I felt the wind under my outstretched arms as I flew. The eagle was taking me on a guided tour. We were flying high over snowcapped mountains; I recognized them as part of the Rocky Mountains chain. We swooped and swirled with gusts of wind. We dived down close to the mountains, then rose again, riding the currents.

I felt so free! Who wouldn't want to leave a body where you can't put one foot in front of another? Who wouldn't want to fly effortlessly, carried along by gentle breezes?

Suddenly, the scene changed. I was no longer an eagle. I was walking hand-in-hand with another woman on a hiking trail. We stopped and held each other for an indeterminate amount of time. Just holding, just communicating without words. Then as quickly as it started, the astral flight landed. I came back into my body.

This was the only astral trip I have ever experienced. It was a stark contrast to my daily life. Because I cannot feel my legs, I cannot stand. If you cannot stand, you cannot hug someone with your whole body. Stop for a minute and think about it. Most people take for granted the ability to hug a friend or a partner. I can't do that. How many hugs have I missed out on my entire life? Quite a few!

Not being able to walk changes the dynamics of being with a partner. Usually, partners take turns doing things, everything from household chores to going to the store.

"It's your turn to get up and put the DVD in the player," Kirie jokes. "I did it last time."

"Yes, and the time before and the time before that. You know I'm just pretending to be handicapped so I don't have to help out. When you fall asleep, I get up and walk around the house."

"I know you do. Some night I'm going to catch you and the gig will be up."

One way to deal with reality you cannot change is through humor. In all honesty, people take a lot for granted. Because my hands are numb, I can no longer experience the pure joy of touching another body. I used to revel in the sensory feedback that occurs during lovemaking. I miss it.

Years ago, I used to wonder whether my sensory deprivation would become so extreme I would no longer be able to enjoy being touched. Thankfully, my mind has taken over where my body left off. It sometimes hurts to be touched so my partner has to be understanding and I have to be willing to communicate. However, by hooking into the energy of my partner and with her gentle touch, my body responds with incredible orgasms. I feel truly blessed that my disease has not taken away the ability to enjoy intimacy. If I could teach other women how to achieve satisfaction through energy and light touch, I would be a millionaire! It is amazing when you can open yourself up to the flow of energy.

Many people have misconceptions about sexual intimacy if you are disabled. Perhaps my next book will be about the experience of achieving and appreciating it. I firmly believe God gave us the gift of intimacy with another human as a pathway to intimacy with the Divine Energy. If you are able to merge with another person on this plane, you can connect with God. I believe while some people have an extraordinary intellectual connection with God or their higher power, my connection is both intellectual and emotional.

Experiencing the merging of souls helps me to understand and experience immersion into the essence of God. If you have never read it, read the *Song of Solomon* or *Song of Songs* as it is sometimes called. It is a biblical description of intimacy at the highest level. Because the discussion of sex makes many people uncomfortable, they prefer to read this short book only as a metaphor. Personally, I believe it is intended to be read at both levels, literally and metaphorically.

Songs have been inspired by the words: "Let him kiss me with the kisses of his mouth, for your love is better than wine." *Song of Solomon 1.2*

"I am my beloved's and my beloved is mine." *Song of Solomon 6.3*

Does this describe intimacy with your partner or with God or both? You decide.

Coming Home to Myself

In March of 2012, I attended my first Shabbat service. Everything about the service resonated with me especially the joy and celebration. All the cells of my body seemed to repair themselves and reconnect after having been fractured and splintered when I was 17. I could actually feel the cellular transformation take place within my body. I'm not sure whether it is Judaism itself that I am drawn to, or if it is the congregation and the rabbi who resonate with me. I resonate deeply with the joyous Judaism of the "unaffiliated" Sedona Jewish community. We are an eclectic group of members ranging from Orthodox to Conservative to Reform, Reconstructionist, Renewal and even some atheists. Watching the rabbi sing and dance down the aisle to *Mi Chamocha* is a magical experience. Every member of the congregation joins her in song, smile, rhythmic clapping and sometimes following her in dance. The excitement and magic are palpable.

While I was exploring New Age philosophy, I learned to hook into another person's energy and experience walking even when my legs no longer worked. I learned to feel the sensation of standing even when I could no longer bring myself to a stand.

I explained all of this one day to the rabbi who, in her younger years, was a ballet dancer. "Do you realize I can hook into your energy when you are dancing down the aisle and actually feel as if my body was dancing?"

"That's wonderful," she responded. "Feel free to dance with me whenever you want to."

"I like doing it because I was never a good dancer. You are so graceful, I get to feel what it would be like to be a truly graceful instead of a klutz."

Sometimes as she starts down the aisle swinging her guitar and two-stepping, she catches my eye and we dance together. I am transported energetically into the dance of joy and praise for the freedom from slavery.

During the conversion process to Judaism, I had the privilege of leading the Torah study of *Acharei Mot* and *Kedoshim*. I deliberately chose to lead this parsha (portion) of the Torah. I had to confront the passage in the Bible that devastated me so long ago – "homosexuality is an abomination against God."

I researched the original Hebrew – *toevah** - which is translated as abomination in the King James Version of the Bible. I confronted the fundamentalist Christianity segment of the population that still uses this passage to shame and humiliate the LGBT community in the name of God.

Even though I didn't want to make the Torah study about me, I did bring up my experiences prior to the discussion of same-sex marriage. I struggled and prayed a lot about it before I chose to talk about my experience. For any gay or lesbian person, especially someone who came out in the early '60s and '70s, it was a time of intense persecution. Coming out first to myself and then to family and friends took a lot of courage, especially 50 years ago. It was, in fact, often dangerous to do so. While society's attitudes have changed somewhat in recent years, young people still struggle with sexual identity issues.

In the end, it was healing for me to lead this portion. When one of my caregivers came in Saturday night after Torah study, he asked "Have you done something to your face? It looks great. Did you do something different?"

"Um, no."

Sunday morning a different caregiver came in. "What have you done your face? Did you get a facial?"

"Actually, no." Spiritual facial? The ironic part is the fact that I did have a facial scheduled for Friday and it got rescheduled for the following Friday. What's different in my face after Torah study? No idea. Maybe the release of the last vestiges of guilt that I didn't even realize were still there. I was finally free of the shame and humiliation that had dogged my path for 50 years.

The Hebrew word "to'evah" (translated "abomination" and "detestable act") is a cultic, not a moral, term. The English "abomination" means abhorrent, loathsome, unspeakably bad. To'evah means ritually unclean. Eating pork is to'evah; having sex with a menstruating woman is to'evah. You cannot come to worship after doing these things until you have been purified.

It is my understanding that the word to'evah and admonition to the Israelites was to refrain from the sex slavery so prevalent in other cultures at that time. Both males and females were kept as sex slaves for their masters. The masters exercised power over their slaves, controlling the lives of the slaves through the difference in status. Just as worshiping idols was prohibited, so was the practice of sex slavery. From that perspective, it is not an admonition about homosexuality as much of that is about sex slavery.

Whew! What a difference a correct translation makes. Too bad those who judge the LGBT community harshly are ignorant of the original meaning of the Hebrew word. In modern times, sex trafficking fits the prohibition in Leviticus; traffickers exercise the prohibited power and control over their victims.

Without Even a GPS

As I was exploring Judaism and deciding to convert, I spent many hours studying Torah, the first five books of the Bible. I particularly liked a portion called Lech Lacha. What struck me about this Torah portion was the fact that Abraham was willing to leave his country, his family. And his way of life without even a GPS to guide him. As I thought about this Torah portion, I wondered how God communicated with Abraham.

Sometimes God does spectacular things like a burning bush, thunder and lightning, making the earth move. As far as I could tell from reading this portion, there was no spectacular display of God talking with Abraham. I tried to imagine what might have happened. Maybe Abraham and Sarah were chatting with the family one night when suddenly Abraham heard God's voice in his ear. Maybe God told him in a dream. Maybe, without any foreshadowing, Abraham suddenly knew in his soul what God wanted him to do.

Like so many things in the Torah, we are given no definitive answers. Sometimes we wrestle with what it means and can only see it through our own eyes and our own experience. And maybe that's why it's written that way… so we can fill in the gaps from our own perspective. After all, if a book is to survive the test of time, it has to leave some room for continual interpretation.

Somehow, God communicated to Abraham that He wanted him to go on a journey. Leave his country. Leave his familiar house. Leave his family. Leave his way of life. He wasn't a poor man so he wasn't leaving homelessness. He was leaving behind a comfortable life. If I were Abraham, I might have asked, "God, why don't you pick someone younger? Someone with more energy and more years left to fulfill the mission." Depending on interpretation, Abraham was at least 75 years of age at the time that he began his journey.

Sounds like a reasonable alternative to me. Then again, Abraham may have said, "God, I'm comfortable here. I would like to live out the rest of my days here. Don't you have a backup plan? Can't someone else fulfill this mission?" Because I don't always have Abraham's ability to see the big picture, I might have tried to bargain with God.

From my reading of this Torah portion, Abraham prepared for his journey and left, without a GPS, without even a map. He trusted God. Have you ever stopped to wonder what would have happened to Judaism or even Christianity if Abraham hadn't taken that leap of faith? Abraham and Sarah would not be our ancestors. We wouldn't be acknowledging them in our prayers and chants. Would God have chosen someone else? Was there anyone else willing to take that leap of faith? At a time in history where people were worshiping idols and pagan gods, was there another person who could have been chosen? How would the single decision of one person, Abraham, have changed history as we know it?

Anyone who knows me knows that I am a Debbie Friedman fan. When the rabbi mentioned our 11th commandment, my first thought was "my 11th commandment is to make my life a blessing." I guess I can blame Debbie Friedman for that one - so much time listening to her music. Debbie has put the story of Abraham to music L'Chi Lach (the feminine form of Lech L'cha.) Words from her songs often echo in my head. I never was able to meet her but I have always felt I knew her. She passed at the age of 59 of a neurological disorder similar to multiple sclerosis. We had a lot in common.

Lech Lacha - I had always interpreted this to mean "go forth." That is not necessarily a bad interpretation. According to the rabbi, it technically means "go into yourself" or "go to yourself." For each of us, the journey is different, but the destination is the same: to learn to love ourselves and those around us. To find ourselves. So how do I make my life a blessing?

As I have wrestled with this, I have realized it takes three things:

1. Willingness to listen to that still small voice somewhere within my soul and listen intently;

2. Willingness to get off my duff and do something about it; and

3. Developing the discernment to know how to approach the mitzvah (good deed). Wrestling with this question has changed my perspective. I can't sit back and wait for mitzvot* to come to me – I have to make the effort to go out and seek them. To go out and see where I can make a difference.

I will give you an example. As I came out of the bank one day, a man was standing on the corner with a sign "RV impounded. Suffering." My immediate response was to rush into judgment; I know vehicles get impounded when you're picked up for a DUI. I have real difficulty with alcoholism. I talked it over with Tina (my caregiver at the time) and she mentioned other reasons vehicles might get impounded – like it broke down and, without the money to fix it, the RV was impounded by the police because it was a traffic hazard. Sometimes, even doing a mitzvah involves discernment. I am learning not to rush into judgment when people need assistance.

On the other hand, on that same day we were coming up to that same intersection – the busiest in Sedona with Walgreens and the bank and the turnoff to Bashas, a local grocery store. As cars followed the green light into the intersection, a little dog darted in and out of traffic. People all around stopped their cars as the dog darted in front of them and crisscrossed through the intersection. Some people got out of their cars and tried to coax the dog to them. For a brief period of time, I saw many people try to save the dog until he found his owner and she scooped him up. I breathed a sigh of relief since my only mitzvah that day was praying for that little guy's safety.

I want to share one other instance of making my life a blessing. I was hiring a new caregiver. Tina had interviewed her and really liked her. Often, I relied entirely on Tina's judgment and did not interview the caregiver myself. For whatever reason, though, I decided to interview the caregiver. We talked for about fifteen minutes. I told her about my upcoming one-year anniversary of conversion to Judaism and about the drash (a talk/sermon in Christian terms) that I would be doing – go to a land that I will show you, a place you do not know. I told her what that meant to me. I told her how I decided to convert to Judaism after the first Shabbat service resonated in every cell of my body.

Tina called this woman the next day to see whether she could come in and start on Friday.

"No, I really appreciate the job offer, but I have decided to go to Minnesota. After my discussion with Marilyn, I have decided my journey means going to Minnesota."

"You're kidding, aren't you?" Tina was incredulous. Who would leave the magic red rocks of Sedona for the cold, snowy winters and humid, mosquito-filled summers of Minnesota?

"I am so grateful Marilyn shared everything with me. She is a true inspiration."

After Tina got off the phone, I couldn't help but laugh. Sedona? Minnesota? Really? I guess everyone has their own idea of the journey – hopefully God won't ask me to go back to a cold climate!

Because this incident had such an impact on me, I texted the Rabbi and asked if she had a few minutes to talk. This was at 10:45 a.m. She texted back that she had an 11 a.m. appointment so she had a few minutes right then.

"You won't believe what just happened."

I told her about my interview yesterday and how the woman was going on a journey to Minnesota as a result of my interview. We laughed about it for a few minutes.

At shortly after 11 a.m., I got a text from the rabbi. The woman who had interviewed with me was her 11 a.m. appointment and she came in to the office with the words "I am on a journey."

The Rabbi walked over and picked up a guitar and sang "L'Chi Lach," the Debbie Friedman song I love. Even though this woman wasn't Jewish and did not know the rabbi, she had apparently made an appointment with her right after leaving my house the day before.

I believe we are all related to each other one way or another. I guess you just never know when your life will touch someone else's. You never know when words you utter will impact another person's life. I do not believe in coincidence. I was meant to interview this woman on that particular day for her particular reason. Life is strange like that. It takes twists and turns you cannot even imagine.

When I graduated from college, I was a physical education major. It is ironic that by the time I was in my mid-30s, I could no longer walk. Thank God I found other means to support myself because a physical education teaching job would have become impossible. When one door closed, another door opened.

*Mitzvot - plural of mitzvah which is an act of human kindness or moral deed performed as a commandment

The Search aka Chronology of the Disease

I'm not a rabbi, a minister, or a guru of any sort. I am simply a person trying to figure out why I am on this earth at this time. If we do, in fact. Choose the time of our birth as New Age philosophy suggests, why now? And if we do choose prior to birth the lessons we want to learn, why did I pick this lesson? Who, in their right mind, would choose to live their life in a chair? Certainly I have questioned this singular philosophy all of my life.

When I was 27 years old, I started to experience symptoms that no one could immediately identify or classify as a disease. My hands would go numb. I would wake up in the morning and shake them, trying to establish more feeling in them. Often, my legs would feel lethargic, if you can imagine a body part feeling a certain way. If legs have emotions, mine were saying "nope, I don't want to." They were throwing temper tantrums like a two-year-old.

Looking back now, I find it ironic I majored in physical education and psychology in my undergraduate work. When I was 27, I liked to work out and would often go to a local community college to run on the track. One day, after my daily run, I stepped into the bathtub, an old clawfoot bathtub, with the accompanying old faucets. I lived in an upstairs apartment in an old part of town where it wasn't always safe to walk at night but the rent was cheap. The bathtub filled slowly, probably due to a lack of water pressure in this old house.

I put my left foot into the tub, waited a couple of seconds and then brought my right foot into the tub. I suddenly realized that the water was scalding hot. I jumped back out of the tub and looked at my left leg. It was red from the hot water up to the level of the water. I then realized my left leg was numb and I hadn't realized how hot the water was. While I had noticed the difficulty with my hands going numb, I hadn't realized that the problem also existed with my legs. This was my first undeniable clue.

My search began for the cause of my numbness. I went first to a local chiropractor because I strongly believe in alternative medicine. I don't like taking pills or undergoing surgery or any other invasive procedure when it is not necessary. Chiropractic helped the symptoms but they did not totally dissipate. I would intermittently experience numbness in my hands and in my feet and legs. I went to medical doctors and had numerous tests for arthritis, lupus, and everything you can imagine. Nothing showed up in the tests other than the fact that I was having neurological problems. I knew they were getting worse, but I was not going to allow the problems to stop me.

I enrolled in Michigan State University to get a Master's in Business Administration. At that point in time, the program was aimed toward students who would be working in Fortune 500 companies. Most of the students were much younger than I was; they had progressed from getting a bachelor's degree directly into the Master's program. Most of them had never had a job even flipping burgers. Because I had already been a teacher, a social worker, and a unit supervisor, I felt like an old lady compared to these young kids!

While I was enrolled full-time in the Master's degree program, I was also working full time managing four chiropractic offices. I couldn't help but laugh to myself when the other students would complain about how hard the program was – they weren't working a job at all. All they had to do was study. I guess I have always felt that I can work twice as hard as most people and that was certainly the case as I worked on my degree. What made this time most difficult were the symptoms I was experiencing. I was going through the exacerbation/remission phase of my disease without having a definitive diagnosis at that point. It wasn't until I graduated and went to the Mayo Clinic that a specific diagnosis provided for my symptoms.

The medical team at Mayo Clinic ran numerous tests including bloodwork, urine tests, neurological testing, CAT scan and brainstem auditory evoked response. After three days of being poked and prodded, I met with a neurologist. He told me what I already knew – they suspected I had multiple sclerosis.

"What do you mean you *suspect* I have it?" I inquired.

"We are 95% certain that is the problem. We would like to keep you over the weekend for a spinal tap to be sure." he responded.

"What would that accomplish?" I wanted to avoid unnecessary testing especially since I had heard about the risks involved in injecting dye into my system.

"It would rule out a brain tumor. That could also cause your symptoms."

"For the 5% chance that you are wrong, I don't think I want to undergo that procedure," I replied.

So I left Mayo Clinic with the diagnosis I had suspected for the last two years... multiple sclerosis. On one hand, it was frightening to get the diagnosis confirmed. On the other hand, at least I had a diagnosis that would explain the ongoing symptoms.

My visit to the Mayo Clinic occurred in the early 1980's. At that time they did not have MRIs to diagnose the disease. It was a differential diagnosis, excluding other things that might be causing the problems I was experiencing. Nowadays, multiple sclerosis is diagnosed with the use of an MRI. Over the next two years, I experienced intermittent exacerbations and remissions. The symptoms would get worse with extreme numbness and difficulty moving my legs. Then they would get better. Every time I experienced an exacerbation/remission cycle, my body never quite returned to its original disease-free self. I continued to have some loss after every exacerbation.

I soon realized that the diagnosis of multiple sclerosis precipitated a grieving process that never quite ends. After each exacerbation/remission cycle, I would experience anger, denial and bargaining. Eventually I entered the acceptance stage to some degree although I have to admit, I never envisioned living the rest of my life in a chair. After all, I was a physical education major. I was a jock. I loved playing golf even though I was never any good at it. I played tennis. I played racquetball. I enjoyed hiking. I even owned a pop-up camper because I loved getting outdoors and camping.

Living with a chronic disease or illness also involves an element of fear. Will it get worse? Will the symptoms recur? What will happen in a few months or a few years?

Like many young people, I had the illusion of invulnerability. It couldn't happen to me. But it did. I don't know why even to this day. Some people say to me "You must have learned patience from this." I can only laugh. No, I haven't learned patience. I have learned tolerance.

As I was learning to accept the disease, I read the book *When Bad Things Happen to Good People*. I didn't realize at the time that it was written by a rabbi. Since I had turned my back on God, where could I go for spiritual solace? A personal connection with God is what makes my 11th commandment potent.

Illusion of Invulnerability

Prior to the diagnosis, I thought I was invulnerable. I think most people live under an illusion of invulnerability – "it can't happen to me" - until it does. I've even heard lawmakers recently indicate that people with pre-existing conditions have caused the problems themselves. While that might be true of certain conditions related to smoking or alcohol abuse, it is certainly not true of every condition. I know I lived under the illusion of invulnerability until this disease happened to me.

When I was getting my bachelor's degree from Central Michigan University, I traveled back and forth between Saginaw where I was doing my student teaching and Mount Pleasant where I was finishing classes. One snowy day, I was riding with a friend who had grown up in Brooklyn. In New York City, where few people learned to drive. Almost everyone takes public transportation to their destination. So my friend Barb was a novice driver even though she was in her 20s. She had never taken driver's education. And, she didn't have experience driving in Michigan winters.

On that day, we were on a two-lane road behind a slow truck. She decided to pass the truck when there was no oncoming traffic. As she was passing, the truck veered into the passing lane somewhat, and she attempted to avoid him. In the process, we hit a patch of black ice. For people unfamiliar with black ice, it is a strip of pavement that looks wet, but is actually icy.

When she hit the black ice, she overcorrected and the VW started to go off the road. I immediately knew we were going to roll the car.

They say your life flashes before your eyes in near-death experiences. I didn't have that flash at all. I just had a sinking feeling in the pit of my stomach as the car started to roll. I grabbed the dashboard with my left hand and held onto the handle above the door with my right. As the car rolled over and over, I knew we were not going to walk away from this accident unscathed. It was too dramatic, too catastrophic. The car finally stopped rolling and landed on the passenger side. The front windshield was knocked out completely.

Surprised that I was still alive, I unfastened my seatbelt and turned to my friend, "Are you okay?" I asked.

She nodded. "I'm okay but I can't move. My weight is against the seatbelt and I can't unfasten it."

I unfastened my seatbelt and then worked with her to get hers unfastened also. We crawled out from the car where the windshield used to be. As we looked up and around, we had rolled over and over in the soft snow. All of the windows of the car had popped out intact about 100 feet from where we were currently standing; I had to assume they popped when we landed on the top of the car during the first roll. I feared the car itself was totally destroyed.

We went to look at the car the next day at the junkyard where it had been towed. No part of the car was left intact. The top of the car was smashed in. Both doors had huge dents. No windows were left at all.

A young man accompanied us to view the car. "Did you know the people? Was it your friends or family?"

At first I didn't understand why he asked the question. Then I realized he thought people had died in the accident.

"It was her car," I replied, pointing to Barb.

"You weren't hurt? I can't believe you survived this crash without injury."

"No, we walked away from it."

Of course, it helped that the soft snow cushioned the blow as the vehicle rolled over and over. While we were both bruised the next day from the seatbelts, neither one of us was hurt in any other way. Were we lucky? Absolutely! I firmly believe the only thing that saved us was the fact that we both had work in this life to finish. Our survival constituted a major miracle.

I Guess They Didn't Like the Food

Later that year between graduating from college and starting my first teaching job, I worked as a waitress in a Big Boy restaurant. One rainy night around 9:30 p.m, we were all watching the clock. We closed at 10 p.m. all the customers had left. Only the manager who served as the cook and two waitresses remained. We were in the process of cleaning off the tables and booths, filling the salt and pepper shakers, replacing the napkin holders and filling the ketchup bottles. We were almost finished when three young black men sauntered into the restaurant.

Instead of grabbing a table or booth, they sat at the front counter and ordered burgers and fries. One of the males looked extremely familiar to me. When I waited on them I almost asked, "Don't I know you from somewhere?"

Since they were all young, it is quite possible I had seen him in the halls while I was doing my student teaching. For whatever reason, I kept my mouth shut and just went about my business of getting everything ready to close up.

I had my back partially turned from the counter when the three males got up to leave. Out of my peripheral vision, I glimpsed the shotgun as it was pulled out from under the jacket of the oldest male. A few seconds later, I felt pressure against my back and heard a click. The youngest of the trio had come around the corner of the counter and was behind me.

I knew he had a switchblade pressed against my back.

Without thinking, I pushed the other waitress ahead of me and glanced at the male with the gun. His partner had pulled out a pistol and they were motioning to the manager to open the cash register and empty it. With the knife pressure against my back, I continued to push the other waitress ahead of me and walked toward the back of the restaurant. In those days, Big Boy restaurants had large walk-in refrigerators to keep their famous strawberries for strawberry pie as well as other perishables. The young man shoved me into the refrigerator and shut the door.

My mind raced frantically. "What is happening?" the other waitress asked.

"We are being robbed. The guys at the front are making the manager empty the cash register."

"What can we do?"

I shook my head. As I looked at the shelves in the refrigerator, there were boxes of strawberry filling, shelves of bread, gallons of milk, hamburger buns. Nothing to stop a bullet. Nothing to defend ourselves. I pushed the cart containing bread over to the door. I knew it wasn't any protection but it was the only thing that we had.

"They have to kill us," I announced. "We can identify them. They sat at the counter and ordered. They can't let us live."

When I looked at her face, I realized I shouldn't have spoken the words that were in my mind. While I was facing the reality, she was scared to death. We were defenseless.

After what seemed like hours, and I'm sure it was only a matter of a minute or two, the refrigerator door opened. I was sure we were going to be sprayed with bullets and left for dead. Instead, the manager was shoved into the refrigerator and the door was closed again.

"What happened?"

"They took all the money. He made me give them all the money." The manager's voice was shaking. He was a dark skinned Lebanese man but his face was now pasty white.

"What are they doing now?" I wanted to know. "Did they leave?"

"I don't know," he replied. "I don't know. I don't know." He stood by the door, his black eyes darting back and forth like a deer in the headlights.

We waited in the cold walk-in refrigerator for at least five minutes. Finally, my mind cleared and I realized they had probably left the restaurant right after getting the money.

"Let's get out of the refrigerator and call the police."

"No, no," he protested. "They told me to stay in here. If we leave they will kill us."

"They are not going to be staying out in the restaurant waiting for us to get out of the refrigerator. I'm not even sure they realize that we aren't locked in, that we can open the door."

The manager continued to protest. Instead of listening to his nervous jabbering, I pushed my way past him and opened the refrigerator door. A gentleman was standing at the counter. "Are you still open?" he asked.

"No, we're not. We were just robbed. Did you see anyone when you came in?"

"No, no one was here." He shook his head emphatically.

By this time, the manager had finally peeked his head out from behind the refrigerator door and was heading to the phone. In his broken English, he called the police and reported the robbery.

When the detectives arrived, they questioned each of us separately. The other waitress didn't remember anything and was the first to leave the restaurant. While one of the detectives sat with me in the booth, another detective sat with the manager in an adjoining booth. I could hear the manager frantically describing the situation "the guy had a machine gun. He had a machine gun."

The detective questioning me had a quizzical look on his face. "Did you see a machine gun?" Since this incident happened in the '70s, it occurred before all of the AK-47 shootings.

"No, when he got up from the counter, he pulled out a gun from underneath his jacket. It looked like the shotgun my dad used for hunting."

"A sawed-off shotgun then," he concluded.

"That would be my guess. I've never seen one before but that makes sense."

As we sat in the booth and the detective took my descriptions of the three males, I told him I believed one of them was not even an adult. I thought he was probably 15 or 16 years old. I also told him about the one who had pulled out the shotgun. He was the one who looked familiar to me. I explained that I almost said something about him looking familiar.

The detective shook his head. "Thank God you didn't."

"Why?" That seemed like an innocent question.

"One of two things would've happened," he explained. "Either they would've decided not to rob you in the first place or they would've shot you so you couldn't identify them. It's a 50-50 proposition. In either case, you are lucky you did not say anything. I wouldn't have wanted to take those chances under the circumstances."

For the first time that night, I breathed a sigh of relief. The next day I had to go to the police station and look through yearbooks to see if I could identify the individuals. The police caught them almost immediately and a few months later I had to testify at the trial. I slept with the light on for two weeks before I could finally turn the light off and go to sleep.

I hope the next time a customer doesn't like the food, he or she decides not to leave a tip rather than rob the joint!

Before I ever started my first professional job, I had already had two close calls with death. Was I invulnerable? Was I a cat with nine lives? After each instance, I felt lucky to be alive.

Fired Without Cause

I followed my chosen teaching career for one year and was fired from my first professional position. I taught at a Catholic high school in Saginaw, Michigan. Apparently, I was too liberal. Two members of the senior class scheduled an appointment to talk with the history teacher and me. The young man was concerned because his girlfriend couldn't have an orgasm. We answered their questions honestly. The next day, I was called to the principal's office.

"I understand you talked with two of our students about sex," she confronted me in her sternest voice. "And from what I hear, you did not counsel them to refrain from having sex."

"They were already doing it," I blurted. "It is a little late to say 'don't do it.'" The image of shutting the barn door after the horse was already out came to my mind but I didn't say it.

"It was still your responsibility to counsel them about abstinence. You should not be talking about anything regarding sex education."

"Is sex education being taught here?" I honestly had never heard students talk about sex education from any other classes.

"Reproduction is being taught in Sister's biology class." My mind flashed to high school and college biology classes. I didn't remember being taught human sexuality.

"So she is teaching about human sexuality?" I persisted. To this day, I never quite know when to shut my mouth!

"Of course not," the principal replied indignantly. "She teaches them about frogs and other animals."

In other words, the students were supposed to extrapolate from the animal kingdom and understand sex. Knowing it was an argument I could not win, I got up and walked to the door.

"Do not talk with students about sex again," she cautioned. Apparently, I didn't listen well. Later that year I taught a chapter of human sexuality as part of my psychology class. Whenever students would ask questions I answered honestly. To this day, I think it is important to honor curiosity with straightforward answers.

On another occasion, I went to the principal to inform her that students were smoking marijuana in the bathrooms.

"How can you possibly know that's what they are doing?" She asked in her authoritarian voice.

"Because I smell it when I pass by."

"How do you know what it smells like?"

""Because I just graduated from college," I replied. "Even if I didn't smoke, most of the other students did."

"Well," she huffed. "We do not have a drug problem at this high school. Remember that."

So I left her office feeling chastised for wanting to bring a potential problem to her awareness. Two weeks later, an eighth grade student was visiting for a day as part of an orientation to the high school he would be attending next year. While he was there, he was sold some bad drugs and ended up in the ICU that night.

The next day we had an emergency teacher's meeting. The principal explained what had happened and what she expected from the teachers as a result. "We have a serious drug problem here," she pointed out in a solemn tone. "From now on, every teacher will forfeit lunch hour and patrol the halls and lunchroom. In addition, you must give up prep time to patrol the bathrooms and external grounds. You will be assigned outside or inside duty."

While I sat at the teacher's meeting feeling vindicated, I was still uncomfortable knowing she was not willing to listen to me initially.

That year, all of the lay teachers were fired except one. Even one of the nuns who was fired because she fraternized with one of the male teachers too much. They would sit and talk in the art room after school; I didn't know it was possible to fire a nun, but that is what happened!

I licked my wounds for a few days. How humiliating to be fired from my first professional job! After that, I left Michigan and went to Jacksonville, Florida where I was hired to work for the state in the Division of Retardation. To be politically correct, they have now changed the name to Office of Developmental Disabilities.

In any case, I was no longer a teacher. I had become a social worker.

Another Brush with Death

Part of my responsibilities as a social worker was to make home visits and assess the needs not only of the client but also of the family. The city of Jacksonville, Florida is also the entire county. To my knowledge, it is the only city that is also an entire county. The city itself is divided by a river. Most of the homes on one side of the river were in the residential areas with groomed yards and upscale neighborhoods. On the other side of the river were federal housing projects. Many of our clients lived in federal housing projects that were known to be somewhat violent. In the worst project, the fire department would not respond to a call without a police escort. Social workers, however, were expected to go into the project unarmed and unprotected.

A few days before Christmas, another social worker and I were making a home visit to a client who needed daycare for her developmentally delayed 3-year-old. As we walked into the Blodgett project at 8 a.m., we met two young teenage males. I don't make eye contact usually under those circumstances but I did watch them peripherally. I had the eerie sensation something bad was going to happen… like watching a car accident happen before your eyes. I kept walking nevertheless.

We had only walked about 50 feet more when I felt a push from behind; one of the young men was grabbing my purse while the other young male was pushing me down. I couldn't fight the two of them. I screamed at the top of my lungs just before I hit the ground with my mid back slammed against the side of the sidewalk. They ran off with my purse. As I got up off the ground, I noticed that a number of doors were opening and people were standing in the doorways.

"Stop them," I yelled. "They stole my purse."

As I looked around at the people standing in the doorways, I was met with blank stares. Then, the doorways closed and the residents went back inside one by one. The other social worker with me gave me a surprised look.

"What happened?"

She was oblivious to the whole event; I had known she was scatterbrained but really? She had no idea why I was suddenly slammed to the ground.

"Billie, they stole my purse. Let's get the hell out of here."

"We still have to make the home visit," she persisted.

I just stared at her with a dumbfounded look. "I'm getting the hell out of here," I declared. "If you want a ride, you will come with me."

I turned quickly and started marching out of the project. Eventually, she caught up with me.

"What are you going to do?"

"I'm going to report this to the police," I responded. "But I doubt I can recognize them or identify them in a lineup. It's a lost cause, I'm sure."

When we got back to the car, I mentally thanked the social worker who had originally trained me. She taught me to put my purse over one shoulder and hold my car keys in the opposite hand. Because of that small training tip, I was able to immediately exit the housing project and get to safety. Of course, I had to replace all of my identification and credit cards but they didn't get my car.

When I returned to the office, I reported the incident to my supervisor. Because I had been slammed against the sidewalk hard, I visited the doctor and was given pain pills for my back and a couple of days off. I can't say for sure but I think the trauma to my back precipitated the onset of the MS. In all of the reading I have done, many individuals with MS have reported a fall or accident that occurred prior to the onset of symptoms. It was after this trauma I started to experience numbness and tingling of my arms. I attributed it to the spinal trauma but maybe that wasn't the full cause of the problem.

Prior to the diagnosis of MS, I had three close brushes with death.

Invisibility

By the time I was 35, I was spending the majority of my day in the wheelchair or power chair. Walking had become increasingly difficult and I had to use a walker or hold onto the wall to maintain balance. Associated with multiple sclerosis, fatigue poses a common problem and rears its ugly head frequently. I used the chair so I could remain productive during the day. At this time, I learned what it was like to be invisible.

One day I went to a clothing store to get a new suit for a seminar I was conducting. When I approached a clerk to ask about the dressing rooms, the clerk looked over my head to the friend who accompanied me and asked "Would she like to try them on?"

My friend answered. "Why don't you ask her? She has ears, you know. She can't walk but she can hear."

The woman blushed and led us to the dressing rooms. Without any type of Star Trek cloaking device, I had become invisible.

On other occasions, people would come up to me and talk in a very loud voice. Apparently, if you are using a wheelchair, people assume you cannot hear them. What I found most prevalent, however, was the fact that most people would just simply glance and look away quickly in embarrassment. I actually grew to appreciate the people who would look me in the eye and say "You look so healthy. Why are you in the chair?"

I appreciated the fact that they could acknowledge me without diminishing my dignity. Whenever I was approached with that type of question, I answered honestly. As a society, we seem to feel more comfortable with people being disabled when they are older. Disability at a young age seems to lead to others' discomfort.

One day in the grocery store, a little boy of about four or five years of age was following me around and pointing at me. His mother would sheepishly pull him away and shush him up. He persisted. He continued to follow me around and point at me. Unbeknownst to me, my dog was sitting on my feet. Whenever I was working, she would crawl up onto my feet, curl up, and fall asleep. On that particular day, she was still sleeping on my feet when I went to the grocery store. The little boy wasn't pointing at me, he was pointing at my dog. When his mother finally realized what was going on, she came over to me, "That's so cute that your dog is taking a ride with you."

I looked down. Sure enough, Skunk, my Shih Tzu, was riding around on my feet. She sat up, acknowledged the little boy and laid back down.

"Thanks for letting me know. I didn't even realize she was taking a riding along."

I grew to appreciate the honesty and curiosity of kids. They don't judge. They just ask questions. I never really noticed Skunk was there until she died and was no longer lying on my feet. Then I missed her acutely.

Along with invisibility, I have other pet peeves related to my disability. Nowadays, too many people are taking advantage of the movement toward service dogs, pets who actually serve a critical physical and/or emotional purpose for disabled people. They buy a scarf and put it on their dog so they can take them to the grocery store or to the restaurants even though the person isn't disabled and the dog is not a trained assist dog. To those people who really need and use a dog to mitigate the effects of their disability, it is a slap in the face.

From the perspective of someone who is disabled, it is similar to the use of handicap parking spaces by people who are able-bodied. They have no sticker. They have no disability. When I have watched an able-bodied person get out of the car after parking in a handicapped spot, I have left notes on the car "When you park in a handicapped spot illegally, you are asking God to make it legal for you. Think about it. Is that what you really want?"

I have heard the excuse "I'm only going to be five minutes. I just have to pick up a few things." During that five minutes, I might be sitting in the hot van waiting for the handicapped spot to open up. Because people with multiple sclerosis are extremely heat sensitive, your lack of consideration can make me miserable and render my body dysfunctional.

I attended a local movie theater recently. Only two handicapped spaces were available and one curb cut that allowed handicap access to the sidewalk. A Porsche was parked so it totally blocked the curb cut out. My partner went into the movie theater and asked that the car be moved so I could get into the theater.

A man spoke up and said, "I will be moving it in a minute. I just had to drop off some things for the theater."

Five minutes later, the car was still parked firmly in front of the curb cut. Again, my partner went in and asked that the car be moved and complained to management. After another five minutes, the guy came out and shouted as he got into his car, "What is your big problem?"

With a look of absolute disgust, my partner replied, "You. Your total lack of consideration for someone who truly needs a handicap parking spot. Hopefully karma will render you deserving of this spot in the future." No excuse for absolute rudeness.

Situations like this infuriate people who truly need handicap parking and curb cuts. No able-bodied person has a good excuse to park in a handicap spot merely for their own convenience or with the excuse they will only be there for a few minutes. I sometimes wish I could be Tuwanda from the movie *Fried Green Tomatoes*. I could shove their car out of the way with the caveat "I'm older and I have better insurance!"

This past weekend I went to a dinner club show at the Blazing M ranch. Dinner is served at picnic tables inside a big barn-like atmosphere. After dinner, local talent is featured in the show. When we sat down at the table, a woman we'd never met was sitting opposite us. She turned to Kirie.

"What do you do?"

"I am retired now. I used to own and manage a woman's campground."

"Oh my God, that would be so much fun. That would be an awesome experience."

"It was," Kirie acknowledged, "until the redneck neighbors decided to try and hassle my campers. I had to take out my shotgun and shoot over their heads to get them to leave the property."

"I can't imagine what that was like."

"Owning the campground was a lot of work but I enjoyed it. I didn't enjoy having to keep the neighbors in line. Because we were out in the country, it would often take 30 to 45 minutes for the sheriff's department to respond to a call. I had no choice but to protect the property."

"That must've been difficult," the woman agreed.

After the show I realized that while I had asked her profession, she never inquired about mine. She never found out I own two businesses, and even though I am in a wheelchair, I still work and contribute to society. That's what I mean about being invisible.

I have also experienced the opposite extreme from invisibility, people violating my personal space by using my wheelchair to lean against while I'm waiting in line at the grocery store. Just like any other person, my personal space extends three feet around me including my chair. It is intrusive and a violation of my personal space when people use my wheelchair as their leaning post. I am not invisible. I don't want to be treated like I can't be seen. Invisibility takes many forms.

Why Can't I Stand?

While I was in my 40's, I decided to join the Michigan Athletic Club so I could use its pool to work out. Two or three times per week, I went down to the club with my caregiver. Because I couldn't stand, I couldn't change my clothes after getting in the pool. Imagine leaving the club in zero degree weather wearing wet clothes and getting into a cold van for the 10-minute trip home. Not fun! I was determined to maintain as much strength as I possibly could and not lose muscle mass.

To achieve my goal, I decided to hire a personal trainer to work out with me three days a week. Todd was 220 pounds of pure muscle. He was an Ironman competitor and a great trainer. As part of the workout, I would lie flat on my back on a table and he would put my feet against his chest. While he held onto the edge of the table, I pushed as hard as I could against his chest.

"I can't believe how strong your legs are," he remarked one day. "I am working with seven other people with MS and none of them is nearly as strong as you are. During your next session, we are going to try to get you to stand."

"Sounds good to me."

I had a standing wheelchair that I used for workouts three or four times a week. With the wheelchair, my legs were locked in place so they couldn't buckle.

At our next session, I pulled my chair up to a railing. With both hands gripping the railing and his hands underneath my armpits, I tried to pull myself to a stand. Despite pulling with my arms, pushing with my legs and having his assistance behind me, I couldn't come to a full stand.

Frustrated, he said, "I don't get it. You have more strength than anyone else I'm working with, and yet you can't stand. Three of my other clients are able to walk. Why can't you?"

"I wish to hell I could answer that. Honestly, I can't feel my legs. They feel like wood. They don't feel like they belong to me. I can't tell if they are under me or not."

"I know my other clients say their legs feel funny. Can you describe it in more detail?"

"Not really. Other than to say that they feel disconnected and not part of my body, I don't know how else to describe it. I really can't tell if I'm standing or not."

"Okay, I'm going to brace your legs from behind. Can you lock your knees?"

With Todd bracing my legs and helping me maintain my balance, I was able to stand for about five seconds. Or at least that's what he told me. From my perspective, I still didn't feel like I was standing. I honestly couldn't tell.

During this time, I was working with an energy healer. She would pull energy from Mother Earth and transfer it to my body by laying on of hands. Many times I could actually feel the energy as it buzzed through my body. During one of my workout sessions, she accompanied me to see if running energy as I attempted to stand would make a difference.

With Todd behind me, she ran energy and braced my knees from the front. With both of them working with me, I still could not lock my knees and stand for any period of time. It was not a matter of having enough strength. The neurons would not fire sequentially due to the damage caused by MS. Because the myelin sheath that protects the nerves is damaged by multiple sclerosis, the nerve impulses just don't travel the way they should. All of the strength in the world did not make enough of a difference to allow me to stand.

Living Alone Has Its Hazards

As the MS progressed, I found it necessary to hire caregivers to help with my daily activities. I usually had someone come in for a few hours every day. With a lift in a handicapped van, I could still get out and shop for myself initially. On one occasion, I went to the local grocery store. While I was shopping, the outside temperature rose dramatically. After the groceries were put in my van, I drove my scooter into the van and attempted to transfer to the driver's seat. Because MS is extremely heat sensitive, I became overheated quickly and couldn't make the transfer. With the windows of the van closed, I tried to get someone's attention. I finally caught the attention of one of the baggers, but he tried to ignore me. I hollered louder. Finally he came over to the van.

"Please help me transfer into the car seat."

Catching his look of disdain, I felt humiliated and embarrassed. He turned and tried to walk away. I hollered again. "Please help me!"

He slowly turned back toward me. When he came over, he exclaimed "I don't know what you expect me to do." His attitude was one of exasperation and indignation.

"I can tell you what I need. Please come into the van and help me."

Remember, this was over 20 years ago when we didn't have cell phones. I couldn't reach the horn on the steering wheel. Imagine the loss of dignity when you have to plead for assistance and you have to learn to swallow your pride.

I know that dealing with handicapped people can intimidate some people. For him, I was definitely an inconvenience. For me, I had no choice. The longer I sat in the hot van without being able to transfer to the driver's seat and turn on the air conditioning, the worse I felt. After explaining what I needed, he was able to help me get into the driver's seat. When I returned home, I sat in the van for twenty minutes with the air conditioning on high so I could cool my body enough to get out. Few things are worse than feeling helpless and having to ask for help for even the simplest things.

Most people are able to maintain independence until advanced age takes over. I lost my independence while I was still in my 30's. I learned to ask for help when I couldn't reach things on grocery shelves. I learned to ask for help when I couldn't pick up something from the floor I had dropped. And if no one was available to ask, I simply learned to do without or wait until someone was available.

When dealing with increasing disability, situations arise where you have no control. One day, I was getting into the van from my driveway. My scooter was part of the way onto the ramp and the ramp started to lift on its own. I don't know why. With my front wheels on the ramp and my back wheels on the driveway, my scooter flipped backwards and threw me to the ground. At that point in my life, I could still pick myself up, manage to get the scooter upright and get back onto the scooter. Needless to say, I was so rattled and frustrated that I didn't attempt my trip for the day. I just went back in the house.

On another occasion, I was coming home from visiting a friend. One problem with MS is that you either have to go to the bathroom or you don't. And when you have to urinate, the need is urgent. There's not a lot of warning. On that occasion, I was fumbling with the keys to my front door and couldn't get it unlocked. Because I had to go to the bathroom really badly, I ended up peeing in my jeans. I was probably only 35 at the time. Usually, people don't have problems with incontinence until they are in their 50's or 60's at least. I had to give up part of my dignity at a much earlier age.

During my late 40's, I was still attempting to live alone. It was becoming increasingly difficult. Even the simplest tasks would wear me out. One time as I reached under the kitchen sink to turn on the garbage disposal, I lost my balance. I started to slip out of the chair and frantically grabbed for the countertop to push myself back in. That didn't work. Slowly I slipped out of the chair and onto the kitchen floor.

As I went down, my right eye came to rest against a drawer handle. With as much strength as I could muster, I pushed myself away so the handle didn't pop out my eye. In the process, the rest of my body slid to the floor. My scooter was behind me wedging in my legs so they couldn't move. My head was tilted at a 90° angle so I could barely breathe. I couldn't move. I was totally stuck.

Because I was always concerned about safety, I was wearing a lifeline. I reached my hand up carefully and pushed the button. It fell apart in my hand and dropped to the floor. I probably should have felt panic at that point; instead I felt in eerie sense of calm. It was Friday night. Monday was July 4. None of my caregivers were due to come in until Tuesday, July 5. As far as I could tell, the lifeline didn't work and did not call anyone.

While I'd had several brushes with death, this particular occasion hit home hard. I was going to be alone for four days. My lifeline had broken and lay in pieces underneath me. I couldn't move my legs to get in a more comfortable position. With my head tilted at a 90° angle against the drawer, breathing was difficult and if I relaxed my neck even a little, I couldn't breathe. The extreme angle of my neck literally cut off my windpipe.

As I lay motionless, I realized I would probably lose my ability to hold my head up so I could continue to breathe. When that happened, I would lapse into unconsciousness. My only prayer was, "God, if this is my time to go, please do not let it be painful." I was not scared. I didn't feel fear. I was at peace.

After approximately 45 minutes, I heard someone opening the front door. Apparently the lifeline had worked and had called one of the people on my call list. Jackie rushed in with her partner, Bernie.

"Oh my God! What happened?" she exclaimed.

With the help of Bernie, they attempted to move my scooter. Even with the two of them working together, it took a few minutes to move the scooter enough so I could stretch out my legs. Then they gently helped me get into a lying position on the floor.

"What happened? Are you okay?"

Jackie and Bernie hovered over me. I obviously wasn't bleeding. I didn't feel as if I had broken anything.

"I just bent over to turn on the garbage disposal. I lost my balance. I tried to grab the countertop but I couldn't hold on. Because my face ended up against the handle of the drawer, I was afraid I was going to pop out my eye."

"Are you hurt?" she asked. "Do you need to go to the hospital?"

"No, I don't think so. I didn't break anything. My neck hurts a lot from being jammed against the drawer but I think it will be okay."

Jackie picked up the pieces of my lifeline. She pushed the button. As far as we could tell, nothing happened. A few minutes later, an ambulance pulled up. The paramedics checked me out and wanted to take me to the hospital for x-rays. I declined. Instead, Jackie and Bernie helped me get into my chair in the living room and stayed with me for a couple of hours. When I saw my acupuncturist at the next visit, she observed. "Your neck feels like it has been broken."

"I know it wasn't. I didn't fall and hit it. I know the vertebra are intact."

"That may be," she confirmed. "On the other hand, you have an extreme amount of ligament, tendon and muscle damage. Your soft tissue is a mess."

Even though I received acupuncture and chiropractic care for the injury, my neck ached so badly I couldn't lift my left arm. After two years of extreme pain, I lost the use of my left arm not because of multiple sclerosis but because of the injury.

I write about this experience only because it illustrates how helpless and lonely living alone can feel. I didn't think my lifeline had worked when I pushed it since it fell apart in my hands. I wasn't expecting anyone to come to my rescue for four days. By that time, I knew I would be dead. I could not possibly stay awake and hold up my neck such an extended period of time. My two little dogs were great companions but not able to help in emergency situations.

People have asked if I wasn't afraid when I was living alone. Of course, the answer is affirmative. I knew I couldn't defend myself if someone broke in. Because cell phones weren't invented then, I kept a portable phone near me hoping I could reach it if necessary – and if I hadn't forgotten to charge it! I slept with it and a flashlight under my pillow. But in all reality, I was literally a sitting duck. It gave all new meaning to the phrase.

Setting Your Intentions

Many of the self-help and New Age philosophy books discuss setting intentions and surrounding yourself with positive affirmations. When I left Sedona after a week of vacation, I set the intention "someday I will live here."

It took 15 years to actualize my intention. When I turned 50, Michigan was in the midst of a horrendous winter. For six months, we had no sun. Snow piled high on sidewalks. If I attempted to go anywhere, I was often blocked by snow being shoved into the curb cuts. That particular winter, the mailbox could not be kept clear because the salt from the roads had melted three feet of snow into ice. It literally took a pickax to clear the mailbox for mail delivery.

When we arrived in Sedona, the March weather was gorgeous. Low 70's during the day, low 50's at night. Prior to arrival, I had been working with a healer from Sedona who suggested I spend time outside in the sun even if I was bundled up.

"Thomas, you don't understand," I tried to explain. "There is no sun. We haven't seen sun for months."

"Go outside and sit even if it's cold," he insisted.

"Really, there is no sun. I cannot sit in something that does not exist!"

When I met Thomas, I understood his insistence. He had only lived in California and Arizona. He had never lived in snow and had no idea what it was like to experience months of dreary winter. Sedona experiences over 300 sunny days per year; by contrast, Lansing, Michigan experiences just over 100 days if you count partly sunny days. He could not imagine weeks and months without seeing the sun.

We had only been in Sedona for a couple of days when we went down to Red Rock Crossing. My partner at the time, Berta, had twisted her ankle prior to leaving on vacation. She took off her shoes and walked for a brief time in the cool water of Oak Creek. The next morning we were reading the local newspaper before setting out for the day.

"My foot no longer hurts," she exclaimed as I watched her twist her ankle from side to side.

"Oak Creek has healing properties. That could be why."

"I had a dream last night about moving here," she ventured. "I saw three fingers in a mountain and I saw us finding a place here."

"What are we going to do with the house back in East Lansing? We can't afford both."

She shook her head. "I don't know. I didn't think I would like it here because it's not green like Michigan. But it's a lot greener than I expected. And I really like the weather."

Since I held the local paper in my hand, I looked in the classified section for rentals. Because I need a home that is relatively open and easy to ramp, I wasn't hopeful we would find a home that met our expectations and needs. I was surprised to locate a lease option home in West Sedona. Berta called the landlord and got the address. Since we knew I would be unable to get in the home, she decided to drive there alone to take a look around and check out the neighborhood.

Driving down 89A, the main drag of Sedona, she spied three fingers jutting out from the side of Thunder Mountain. A couple of blocks later, she turned onto the street where the rental home was located. I truly believe there is no such thing as coincidence. Since that day, I have never seen another lease option advertised in the paper.

Getting out of the car, she started looking around the yard. Because she didn't have a formal appointment for a showing, she looked in the front picture window. She was surprised to see a woman staring back at her straight through the house from the back picture window. The woman waved and then came around the side of the house to the front.

"Hi, I'm Vonnie. I live in the house behind. I saw you looking through."

"I can't believe you saw me. We're just looking at the house in case we want to rent it. Do you know anything about it?'

"I know the man who owns it. He's been putting some work into it."

"We are thinking of moving here. I just wanted to check it out."

"It's a good neighborhood. I think you'd like it." With that proclamation, Vonnie took a crystal pendulum out of her pocket.

"Are they meant to live here?" With those words, the crystal started swinging wildly.

"That is a definite yes," she said. "This is your house."

"Are you sure?"

"Absolutely! It swings clockwise for yes. It couldn't be more definite."

We contacted the landlord, saw the inside of the house and made the decision. Until her death, Vonnie was an awesome neighbor and friend. We saw a lot of her crystal pendulum over the years.

We met the landlord and signed the lease. "After looking at all of the bruises on your breasts from the lifting in and out of the plane, I'm going to go back to Michigan and drive the van here," Berta declared. "I'll get the dogs and the bare essentials. I don't want you to have to endure another plane trip."

"Are you sure you want to do that alone?"

"Yes, it's better this way."

Friends and family in Michigan packed up our belongings and Berta returned with the dogs. The book cover is a picture taken at Cathedral Rock, part of Red Rock Crossing. I took my first and only astral trip at that location, flying with the eagles. It's approximately five miles from my house. I go down there often to sit by the creek and enjoy the vortex energy.

Sedona is known for many things. First, it is in the high desert and has beautiful red rock formations. It is like the Grand Canyon turned upside down. In the early 1960's and 70's, many artists settled here. Throughout town, numerous stores sell high-end art. Fair (fare!) warning: Bring your credit card!

In addition, Sedona is famous for vortex energy points throughout the town that have been measured by physicists. If you are sensitive to energy, you can actually feel their effects. Because of the energy draw, it also attracts many spiritual seekers, psychics, and psychic wannabes. My friend, Cynthia Hart, is the reason I first came to Sedona as a visitor. Prior to my visit, she warned me about the wannabes. "Sedona is one of the few places where you can go into the bathroom in a restaurant and emerge with four psychic readings before you have finished washing your hands."

"You mean they're not all like you?"

"Well, I'm either psychic or psychotic. You get to decide."

Because she had already given me a couple of readings, I knew she was truly gifted. She is the real deal. On the other hand, I have met my share of frauds. I was having breakfast in Nick's Westside restaurant one morning when a woman across the aisle started talking.

"Hello, my name is (I have forgotten her name – she made that much of an impression on me.) Where are you from?"

"We live here," I responded.

"Oh, I thought you were probably tourists. I'm surprised you haven't heard about me." She seemed disappointed at our lack of recognition.

"Why should I know about you?"

"I am Sedona's foremost psychic."

I turned and stared at her. "Really? Where do you do your readings?" We seem to have a psychic on every corner here.

She explained her location. "Would you like to schedule a reading?"

I laughed. If she were truly psychic, she could have read my mind.

"You are truly a fraud and full of yourself," I thought. "You don't even have to be a mind reader much less a psychic to know what I'm thinking. My body language itself should tell you."

I politely turned down her offer and went back to finishing my breakfast. Another psychic wannabe ready to prey on the tourists. Not only is it important to set positive intentions, we also have to protect ourselves from less-than-honorable people. Even though Sedona is known for its spirituality, it does have its share of frauds.

Drama of the Day aka Life in a Bubble

Hiring caregivers to help with basic needs is at first humiliating and embarrassing. Once you get past the embarrassment and indignity of not being able to take care of yourself, you then have to deal with the reality. Unfortunately, having caregivers around all of the time changes your life drastically. Because I have been chair-bound for the majority of my adult life, I have had to hire caregivers to help with even the basic daily living skills such as bathing, toileting, cooking meals, and so on. I have been truly blessed because I have been able to generate enough money through my business to pay for caregivers 24/7. What people don't realize is that it costs over $100,000 per year when you need caregivers available all of the time. In addition to the monetary cost, an emotional cost is incurred that no one can appreciate unless they've lived through it. I call it the "drama of the day."

Unfortunately, one of the huge problems with dependency on caregivers is the way that a caregiver's energy impacts an entire household. I have three rules when I hire caregivers: no drinking, no drugs and no drama. Unfortunately, we have experienced problems with all three rules being broken.

For example, caregivers will arrive for a 7 a.m. shift after having closed the bar at 2 a.m. my sensitivity to scents and smells it is so extreme that the smell of liquor on someone's breath or oozing from their pores almost makes me vomit. Not a pleasant thing to wake up to, having someone lean over you with an odor that is nauseatingly offensive.

In addition, it is human nature for people to bring their drama, whatever it happens to be. It would be helpful if people would leave their drama at the door when they enter your home, but that's often not the case.

As another example, fights with their partner often get brought into our home. If it's a typical workplace, the effects are mitigated by all the other energy in an office or retail store or other workplace. However, when the workplace is your own home, the effect is direct and immediate. One of my caregivers got into weekly fights with his partner. When he came into the living room, I could always tell when they had been fighting. He wore his "ugly face," as we used to call it.

"Are you guys fighting again?"

"Yeah, I'm over it. I'm going to move out. I can't stand all of the fights. They are nonstop."

"So, where you going to move?"

"I have no idea. I just threw all of my clothes in the trunk of my car. I will sleep in my car if I have to."

Since this was the 13th time – that I knew of – that they'd broken up, I seriously doubted this was the final straw. You quickly learn not to get involved or take sides in a relationship fight. Inevitably, if you say something negative about the partner, you feel like a fool when they reunite. You have to learn to keep your mouth shut. In my case, I tried to put myself in a bubble so that their fights, their negativity, and their drama did not affect me. That's not easy.

As it turns out, I actually invited him to live in my home for eighteen months until he chose to move out. He was a quiet and respectful roommate.

For other caregivers, we become surrogate mothers. They want to talk about whether to have children, problems with the IRS, their money problems and everything else imaginable. You know how sometimes you just want peace and quiet? You just want to be alone? That's hard to achieve when you have caregivers. If they feel like talking, they intrude on your peace and quiet. Of course, questions always need to be answered, decisions that need to be made, and discussions occur about ongoing projects of running a household. For me, it's even more intense because I run my business out of my home.

Most of the time, I use a headset for my business calls. As a result, my caregivers can hear my side of the conversation if they're listening – and too often they are listening! One caregiver was so nosy she had to make comments every time I got off the phone.

"I would've told them that it's not your responsibility to handle their problems," she said.

"This is my business. I can't tell them that."

"Still, you shouldn't have to hold their hands through everything." She wanted to argue with me about the way I ran my business. Really? Someday I will write a country song "Shut your damn mouth, I don't need your opinion."

Instead I replied as calmly as possible. "You know, this is my business. It is my choice to run it the way I want to. I really don't need your feedback. I've been doing it for the last 30 years without you."

Does that sound rude? Yes, it probably was. But after two or three comments like this, I was totally over it. I don't need a stranger trying to tell me how to run a business I have run successfully for 30 years. Needless to say, she didn't last very long in my employ. She was incapable of keeping her nose out of my business and keeping her mouth shut.

Some people cannot respect privacy at all. Because caregivers are in your home, it doesn't mean you want them necessarily to be part of your family. You want your own privacy and your own life. Whenever I interview a potential caregiver, I talk with them about privacy and the fact that they need to respect our need for space. Some people just don't get that. In another instance, Kirie, her dad and I were watching a movie. That was our family time. The caregiver of the day came into the living room, plopped herself on the couch and proceeded to watch the movie with us. Yes, other chores could have been completed that wouldn't have involved interrupting our family time but, quite frankly, she was lazy. So after plopping on the couch – and taking up the entire couch no less – she enjoyed the movie too much. She was originally from Las Vegas and guffawed at every reference to something specific to her hometown.

The movie was boring; I dozed off. I was awakened abruptly by her loud, raucous laugh.

"You just woke me up," I confronted her in a scolding, angry tone. "Why do you have to be so loud?"

In my head I continued "and why are you sitting here when you should be working?" I didn't say the second sentence aloud even though I wanted to. Needless to say, she didn't last long as my caregiver either.

Privacy when you have 24/7 caregivers is a serious issue. As my partner has said too many times "We live in a bubble. People are always watching us. We can't even fight the way most couples can." It's true. Even if we want to have a serious discussion that doesn't involve disagreement, we have to go into the bedroom and shut the door.

One Sunday morning, we had just hired a brand new caregiver and we needed to talk privately about a family issue. Even though he'd only been in our home for three hours, it became apparent he was in constant need of supervision and guidance.

"We are going in the bedroom for a few minutes." As I looked over at him, he was washing dishes. He gave me a quizzical look but then turned away.

We sat in the bedroom for about thirty minutes as we discussed the issue and came to an agreement. When we left the bedroom, I called his name because I needed his assistance to go to the bathroom. To my surprise, there was a note on the kitchen table. "I understand you need a caregiver but I don't think I'm the one you need. Good luck." He had written the note, signed it and left entirely as we were talking in the other room. Even though we had discussed our need for privacy, it obviously made him uncomfortable. So he just walked out. I didn't even get the opportunity to say "don't let the door hit you on your ass on the way out!"

On another occasion, one of our caregivers decided to quit after only working for a month. He felt a need to confront me as he quit. "Do you mind if I give you some feedback?"

"No, go ahead."

"It is really rude you expect me to disappear and just come whenever you call me."

"You have got to be kidding me."

We have a bedroom in the back of the house where caregivers can go when they're not needed. They can read, watch TV, or do whatever they want. We explain our need for privacy to them when we hire them. He was complaining about sitting on his butt and collecting a paycheck as he was doing it! I was totally taken aback by his comments.

"I am glad you are quitting. I don't need anyone judging my life or my need for privacy."

I clicked the phone off. Because we take great pains to explain our need for privacy, his attitude ticked me off. It is hard enough to have another person's energy always in your home. To have that type of attitude, however, is totally unacceptable. Just imagine having someone always around and then find out he is judging your every communication. Living in a bubble drains energy quickly. He was a definite bubble burster!

When people are constantly in your home, it's difficult not to get sucked into their drama. One of our caregivers opened her home to an alcoholic friend. While she was deer hunting and absent from her house, he bled out on her bed. Needless to say, she was understandably upset and distracted for a couple of weeks.

If a spouse or partner gets sick or hospitalized, that energy is also brought into your home by the caregiver. I often say "drop your drama at the door when you come in," but that's not always possible. If you are sensitive to the energy of people who surround you, it is impossible not to be affected at times. And no matter how hard you try to protect yourself, it drains your energy. Drama that a caregiver brings into your home becomes the "drama of the day." Having lived the majority of my adult life in a power chair, I could write scripts for daytime soap operas just from the dramas we experience on a daily basis.

Physically Challenged?

I suppose as we get older we have more pet peeves. I've listed some such as people parking in handicapped spaces when they don't need it and slapping a harness on a dog as if they are a service dog when they really aren't. I have another pet peeve. Referring to my disability as physically challenged. I know that is supposedly politically correct, but "physically challenged?" If I go to a restaurant, I usually don't order anything to drink because I can't use the restrooms even though they are handicapped accessible. I can't transfer to the toilet.

If I fly in an airplane, I either have to be catheterized or wear a indescribably uncomfortable diaper because I can't stand up and go to the toilet. If I go to the synagogue for the service, we have a wonderful handicapped bathroom – large, grab bars, higher toilet. One of our visitors described it as the Taj Mahal of bathrooms! Unfortunately, I still can't use the restroom so I have to make sure I go to the bathroom before I leave the house. Allowing for drive time and the actual service, I have to be able to hold my urine for at least three hours. Most of the time that's no problem but occasionally it doesn't work out that well for me. I have learned to sit on a disposable pad so I can still enjoy the services without worrying that pee will run down my leg. Personally, I would rather be called disabled or "crip" because this is definitely a lot more than physically challenged. A physical challenge would be climbing Mount Everest!

Performing even the simplest of chores such as bathing, dressing, and toileting are not physical challenges, they are physical impossibilities. For years, I conducted seminars from a power chair. I was conducting a seminar in New York when a chiropractor came up to me during the lunch hour. "I almost didn't stay for the seminar when I realized you were in the chair. When I realized you were the seminar speaker, I almost walked out."

"Why didn't you?" I was curious as to why he decided to stay and didn't walk out at the first break.

"You have changed my perception. I learned more from you in the first two hours than I have learned in any seminar I have taken. I applaud you."

"Thank you very much. I'm glad you decided to stay."

"So am I. I feel much more comfortable going back to my office Monday morning because I know what I'm doing now. You've also helped me realize that a physical disability doesn't necessarily mean you can't learn something from someone."

"I applaud your honesty. Most people are not able to be as honest in their prejudices."

We shook hands and both of us left the room with smiles on our faces.

Because I run a practice management software business, ClinicPro software, I have also had my disability thrown in my face on more than one occasion. When we started selling software in Michigan, we had one main competitor. Often, we would do on-site demos. My competitor would caution people about buying software from my company because I had multiple sclerosis and I was going to die. After I heard that from two potential customers, I called the president of the competing company. "If you do not stop your sales representatives from slandering me, I will sue you. This is not an idle threat. I have heard it from two leads we have both demoed to."

"I don't know what you're talking about," he replied in feigned innocence.

I repeated word for word what the sales representatives were saying. I ended by repeating my caution. "If you do not stop them, I will. I don't mind competition because it makes all of us better. On the other hand, the competition should be based on the products themselves, not on slandering the owner."

They stopped using my disability in their sales pitches. How ironic that the president of that company was deported for a period of time because he had let his visa lapse. I have to admit, I chuckled when I heard about that but I didn't use it in my sales pitches. I like to sleep at night free from guilt.

Because so many of our clients were chiropractors, medical doctors were at first hesitant to buy our practice management software. I remember clearly one day when I demoed to a medical office. I sat in the doctor's office and showed him the program.

After I showed him the complete program, he said, "I like what I see. I think it will serve our needs and be exactly what we need to run my practice."

"Do you have any questions I haven't answered?"

"I don't mean to be rude, but I am concerned about your health. What will happen to your business if you die?" he asked sheepishly.

"I have made plans for business continuation should that happen. We have a support staff who can answer questions and programmers who can continue to develop whatever changes and enhancements you need. Let me turn the tables. What will happen if you die?"

He looked somewhat taken aback by my audacity. "If something happens to me, my practice will die with me."

He bought our software and continued to use it until he retired. As it turns out, he retired and I continue to work. In all honesty, no one knows the date of their death. We all know we have an expiration date, but we don't know when it is.

Self-help books talk about living each day as if it were your last. When you live with a chronic illness or disability, those words ring especially true. Take advantage of every day. Surround yourself with people who share positive thoughts and affirmations because emotional health affects your physical well-being. Don't take yourself so seriously you miss out on opportunities to laugh.

God Doesn't Give You More Than You Can Handle

When people have repeated this adage to me, I have to admit it does anger me at times. I feel like God must have overestimated my ability to handle the challenges of living with disability every day. When people have knee replacements or hip replacements, they have a reasonable expectation they will get up and walk again without pain. I no longer have the reasonable expectation that I will ever walk again. When I try to stand, I cannot feel my legs. They feel like wood. They feel disconnected from my body. They feel like they don't belong to me. And unless you can move your legs to some extent, you can't even roll over in bed by yourself.

One of the hardest things to handle with increasing disability has certainly been the caregivers themselves. I have found it necessary to protect myself from theft of my personal belongings, my medications, my medical marijuana and my sanity!

Because I sometimes have difficulty sleeping as a result of pain, my physician prescribed hydrocodone. I rarely take it but it is good to have on hand if I need it. Shortly after hiring a new caregiver named Terry, I filled my prescription. The bottle had thirty pills. She only worked for less than a month when she quit because "her health was bad."

Because his shop is located on the 2nd floor and inaccessible to me, my hairstylist comes to me. On his next visit, he asked "Where is Terry? I thought she worked for you."

"She did. She only worked for three weeks and then she quit. She said she was having health problems."

He shook his head. "Be thankful she quit. She's a hydrocodone addict."

I checked my hydrocodone bottle. Only four pills were left. No wonder she quit, not much left to steal. I was no longer her drug supplier.

"How did you know?"

"I know her son. Because all the doctors around here know her as an addict, she can't get pills herself. She sends her son to the ER or urgent care to get prescriptions for her."

"For God's sake, why didn't you tell me when you saw her here?" I chastised him thoroughly.

"I didn't want to interfere."

"Come on, that's no excuse. You have known me for years. If you ever know something about one of my caregivers I need to know, tell me."

"I will from now on," he promised.

No matter how thoroughly you perform background checks or attempt to protect yourself, you have no guarantees. Because Arizona has a medical marijuana law, I have a medical marijuana card. For the most part, I have found that a marijuana strain that involves mostly indica works best to settle my muscle spasms at night. For a period of time, my medical marijuana kept disappearing. I finally had to get lockboxes to put my medications in so they couldn't disappear. It's hard to be constantly on the defensive against theft of your medications, but unfortunately that is a reality.

People are addicted to all sorts of drugs nowadays, legal and illegal. If it's necessary to have strangers in your home to care for a loved one, lock up all of your prescribed medications. Otherwise, they may disappear.

Another Commandment Broken

Immediately after a breakup with my partner a few years ago, I had to give a new caregiver the combination to my safe in order to get some documents. A few days later, I got into the safe again. Prior to giving her the combination, I had $500 cash in the safe. It had disappeared. Tina, my daytime caregiver, had been with me for quite a while. She checked and double-checked the safe for the cash. After much discussion, we decided the money had disappeared while the new caregiver was in my residence. We decided to confront the new caregiver as everything pointed to her.

Tina called her. "I'm calling for Marilyn. We have a problem."

"What's happening? What's going on?"

"$500 is missing from her safe," Tina continued. "We know you stole it."

"I wouldn't steal it. I have never stolen anything in my life. It certainly wasn't me who stole it." She protested vehemently for one or two minutes.

"I can tell you for a fact you stole it. We have cameras throughout the house. We have cameras to avoid situations like this. We saw you on camera take it from the safe."

Actually, at the time Tina made that statement, we didn't have cameras throughout the house. We do now. Tina's tone was so accusatory I felt like I had to admit to stealing the money myself! Her accusation was that believable.

The new caregiver started to protest and then stopped. "Yes, you're right. I took it. I've never done anything like that in my life."

"We are going to call the police unless you immediately return the money."

"I can't return it right away. I spent the money on an engagement ring. My fiancé couldn't afford one. So I bought one for myself."

As I listened to the conversation, I found it hard to believe. I allowed her to barter caregiving to work off the money she'd stolen. She ended up quitting for unrelated reasons.

When people steal from you, especially people who you have literally trusted with your life, the betrayal can eat at your soul. It's hard to drop it and move forward with your life. One of my caregivers needed a place to live and I offered him roommate status without rent. He lived with me for over a year. I treated him like my son or grandson. I always thought we were close. When he decided to move out, he grew more and more distant. Some times when he would come in for his shift, he was obviously high. When I confronted him, he told me it was allergies. While I didn't believe him, I hoped he would get his act together. That didn't happen.

One day, my partner went into the back bedroom where the caregivers normally sleep. His backpack was lying open and was stuffed with rolls of paper towels and toilet paper. Since we had just purchased paper towels with prints, she recognized the paper towels immediately. She came into my office to inform me.

"I just saw his backpack open. He is taking paper towels and toilet paper. I don't know why."

I didn't immediately confront him. Instead, I just kept working. He came into my office a few minutes later.

"I want you to know I'm not a thief. My brother asked me to stop at the store and pick up these things and I was going to buy new ones for you later today when I came back in this afternoon." With those words, he went over to the couch and dumped everything out of his backpack.

"See, I have toilet paper and paper towels but nothing else. I will replace them this afternoon. That is what I intended to do."

Obviously, it wasn't about the toilet paper and paper towels. If he had asked, I would have gladly given him the items. I asked him to give me a few hours to think about everything.

I texted him later and asked him to come in for his regular shift the following day. He showed up forty-five minutes late and came into the garage where we were working.

"I quit." He threw the house keys at me and started to walk toward me. His face was angry and menacing. Because she is very protective as a mother hen, Kirie, my partner started to walk toward him. She was going to get between us and defend me physically if need be.

"If you don't intend to work anymore, I need to have the cell phone back." He had asked me to purchase an iPhone for him on my telephone bill. He was supposed to pay me the $750 for the iPhone.

"It's my phone, not yours." He started to walk toward me but stopped when my partner got between us.

"It's really not your phone. You haven't paid me for it. I want it back."

He protested more. "Everything is on this phone. It belongs to me."

"No, it doesn't," Kirie interceded. "If you don't give it back, I will call the police."

With that threat, his face turned slightly white. He did not have a green card and didn't want to have a run-in with the police. He had crossed into Arizona illegally.

"I don't have it with me."

"If we don't have it back within an hour, I will call the police," she responded.

He got in his car and left. He returned thirty minutes later and handed over his phone. He had smashed the front of the phone to make it unusable and had erased all of his contacts. I later learned the truth about my suspicions. He had started using heroin and had become a person I barely recognized.

A couple of weeks later, I went into my safe to show someone the gold lapel watch that had belonged to my great-grandmother. To my surprise it was missing along with a gold buffalo pendant I had commissioned. Only two people other than myself had ever opened my safe and he was one of them. I know the missing items didn't magically fall out of my safe and somehow he'd come up with a down payment for car. I guess I know how. To this day, it breaks my heart because I allowed myself to truly care for him and his well-being.

Perhaps God believes I can handle betrayal but it is extremely difficult when it happens over and over. I have tried to maintain distance from my caregivers for that reason. It's too emotionally draining to get attached in any way and then suffer upheaval of your life as a result.

Dark Night of the Soul

The lyrics of another of Debbie Friedman's songs, *Al Tasteir* taken from one line of Psalm 27, Verse 9:

Don't hide your face from me,
I'm asking for your help.
I call to You, please hear my prayers, oh God.
If You would answer me as I have called to You
Please heal me now, don't hide your face from me.

Many people interpret this line of the Psalm to mean that we have turned away from God and therefore God's face is hidden from us. That is obviously a legitimate interpretation. I interpret it somewhat differently. I feel a kinship with Debbie Friedman even though I never met her. She had paroxysmal dystonia, a neurological disease that mimics the symptoms of MS. According to the documentary film of her life, she woke up one day after a concert the night before and couldn't move her legs. She couldn't get up from bed. Her legs felt like telephone poles. With her neurological disorder, cramping would happen suddenly the more she moved, the tighter her muscles became. If she was tapping her leg to the music, her leg might stiffen and become unusable. I can only imagine the amount of courage it took to schedule a concert knowing that your legs or arms might become unusable in the middle of the concert. Playing guitar when your hand and arm are totally cramped would be impossible. Unfortunately, she died at the age of 59 after a beautifully prolific career of songwriting and concerts.

When you convert to Judaism, part of the conversion process involves immersion in living water called a mikveh, a ritual bath of purity. Because I live in the small town of Sedona and can't get into a traditional mikveh or another source of living water, we performed my mikveh in my swimming pool. Unconventional? Absolutely. I have a ceiling lift that allows me to get in and out of the pool safely. For people unfamiliar with handicap equipment, straps are wrapped under your body somewhat like safety straps you see when people are rappelling down a mountain. A ceiling lift contains a track where a person slides from side to side while suspended in straps.

As the rabbi and I were discussing the ceremony, I remarked I was afraid of water. "I know I drowned in a past life. All my life, even when my arms and legs worked as they should, I've been afraid of water."

"Don't you work out in your pool?" Rabbi Alicia couldn't believe I would actually get in the water and work out considering my fear.

"Yes and every time I do it, I have to summon my courage again."

When I go into the pool, my caregiver puts a noodle underneath my arms and then makes sure I don't pitch headfirst as I work out. It does concern me that I am in the pool alone with someone. What would happen if she suddenly became ill, had a heart attack, or became unconscious for any reason? You don't want to think about those kinds of things, but you have to when you cannot fend for yourself.

Most of the time, my dark nights of the soul do actually happen at night. On two occasions, I have been alone with male caregivers who did not wake up when summoned to roll me. I use a remote doorbell to wake them up. I later found out that one of the guys was addicted to pain medication and therefore slept too soundly to be awakened by my bell. The other guy simply had difficulty waking up. On one of these nights, I had to call 911 because I literally could not rouse him. He was sleeping on the couch in the living room, I was 30 feet away in my bedroom.

"911, what is your emergency?"

"I'm physically handicapped. I can't get out of bed. My caregiver has fallen asleep or is incapacitated and I can't move."

"Have you tried to wake him?"

"Of course. I have rung the buzzer. I have shouted for him."

"Why don't you go and shake him?"

"What is it about the fact that I can't get out of bed don't you understand? I can't walk. If I could walk, I wouldn't need him at all. I believe he is sleeping and I need to get his attention."

After arguing with me for another minute, she finally dispatched the fire department for a well-being check. Just before they arrived, he finally woke up. It is terrifying to be dependent on someone when they turn out to be undependable.

If you can, imagine what it would be like to be helpless and not able to change the situation in any way. That is what I experienced.

No Call, No Show Is No Good

One of the ongoing problems with caregivers is also no call, no show. They literally do not show up and do not call to let you know they're not coming. So as you are preparing for a change of shift, the relief caregiver doesn't arrive. Unless you have someone you can immediately call to fill-in or have family nearby, you are stuck in an untenable situation. Over the years when I have needed caregivers, this has happened at least once a year. In fact, it happened today as I was editing this book. He worked last week for the first time. He was supposed to come in today and simply didn't show up. He didn't call. When you are totally dependent upon caregivers, this is a frightening situation.

One night, I was training a new caregiver. He seemed really responsible and caring so I suggested that Kirie could leave me alone with him even though it was his first night. She has a tendency to stay over when she knows a new caregiver is being trained. I'm grateful that she erred on the side of caution on this occasion. When I rang my remote doorbell that night, there was no response. I rang it three or four times. No response. Finally, Kirie got out of bed and went to the back bedroom. The caregiver was nowhere in sight. He had gotten up and left without even letting us know he was leaving.

"Are you sure he's not out having a smoke?" I asked when she came back into the bedroom.

"I'm positive. Even his car is gone."

"Unbelievable. I am so thankful you are here tonight and didn't listen to me when I said you didn't have to be here."

I hate being a burden on anybody but especially on my partner. It creates a dynamic in the relationship that you really don't want to deal with on a daily basis. I don't want to be dependent on my partner for toileting, bathing, feeding and caring for my daily needs. That's too much to ask.

Today I woke up and rang for my caregiver. I rang my call bell over and over for fifteen minutes. No one appeared. Even though I was alone in the house and in bed unable to move, she decided to take the dogs for a walk. While I admired the initiative, it is unbelievably scary to be alone and unable to move.

Being handicapped takes an obvious physical toll, not only on the person who is handicapped but also on family members who are present on a daily basis. An emotional toll also occurs. There is not only the draining effect of another person's energy in the home, there is also the concern that a caregiver won't show up, might not wake up in the middle of the night, or possibly won't be able to fulfill their duties.

For anyone dealing with a chronic health condition, the dark night of the soul is almost inevitable. It happens. As I often say, "it is what it is." I'm not sure how a person without some sort of belief to sustain them would get through this. I know I have needed a belief in God, Great Spirit, the Universe, or whatever you want to call a higher power to make it through the dark night of the soul.

Unfortunately, it's not just one night. Always looming is the realization that another night can happen at any time, even tonight.

Expect the Unexpected

When I first started to need a power chair, I had one thing I could count on: it would always break right around Christmas time when it was impossible to get service or needed parts. Over the years, I have accumulated numerous chairs so I always have a backup. I estimate I've had at least 15 power chairs, four handicap vans, six ceiling lifts and an untold number of problems with the various mechanics of them. Things happen that are beyond your control.

Because I hadn't been on a real vacation for years, one of my caregivers talked me into taking a road trip to California. My home environment is wonderfully comfortable. I have ceiling lifts throughout the house. I have extra wheelchairs. I have supplies I need for daily living. Trying to conceptualize a road trip and packing everything needed for emergencies was difficult, but I was finally ready to go. As any good business person would do, I scheduled a meeting with a potential client in Los Angeles as part of the trip, combining business with pleasure.

As we traveled, we stopped at a rest area between Arizona and California. When I tried to exit the van, it did not kneel as it should. This type of handicap van kneels so the ramp is not as steep. The kneeling mechanism is a combination of hydraulics and the use of a heavy-duty battery. Since I have had the occasion where the van kneeled and wouldn't go back up, I was more than a little freaked. We certainly couldn't continue the trip to California with the van kneeled or backtrack to my home in Arizona. What to do?

We decided to manually lower the ramp so I could leave the van. Of course, by the time I finally made it into the rest area, I wet myself. We spent the rest of the vacation manually opening and closing the lift because we didn't want to take a chance of kneeling the van and having it stay in a lowered position. Not only do the occupants feel every bump and pothole in a lowered position, it also drags on everything along the road causing damage to the undercarriage of the van itself. It was a nuisance, but manageable.

When we arrived for the first night and had settled into the hotel room, I asked to be put in one of the chairs. My legs were propped up on the coffee table. I asked my caregiver to go to the soda machine and bring me back a can of soda.

When she returned, she handed me my drink, popped hers open and took a gulp. She was standing in front of the loveseat next to me. With a frightened look in her eyes she implored "help me." She slumped to the loveseat with her head lying back.

"What's wrong? What's happening?"

She didn't respond. I called her name. "What's going on?"

I heard a gurgling sound in her chest. I can't really describe it other than it sounded like a waterfall in her chest itself. As I watched in horror, her eyes rolled back in her head.

Needless to say, I became frantic. For years I had resisted owning a cell phone. If I wanted to go out to dinner, I didn't want people tracking me down! Now I wished I'd made a different decision. I looked over at her cell phone. It was lying beside her on the loveseat. No matter how I stretched, I couldn't reach it. Even if I had, I didn't know how to use it to call 911. I was a total newbie.

I looked around the room. There was nothing within reach to help me. I tried to lift my legs off of the coffee table so I could perhaps scooch to the loveseat next to her. For some reason, I had always believed that my legs would work in an emergency. They didn't. They wouldn't budge despite my best intentions.

I glanced back over at her. Her head was lying against the back of the loveseat. Her eyes were rolled back in her head. As I watched, she stopped breathing, her chest was no longer rising up and down.

"Oh my God, her kids. How will I tell them their mom died while I was watching?"

That horrific thought raced through my brain as I thought of her five children, seeing their faces in my head.

"Oh my God, what can I do?"

At that time, I started doing the only option available to me – I started calling her name.

"Allie – can you hear me? Allie, wake up. Allie."

Over and over I called out her name softly, loudly, and then softly again. Her eyes fluttered.

"I hear you." Her soft voice responded after about a minute of constant calling on my part.

"I'm trying to come back." Those words came out haltingly, slowly.

I continued to talk with her for the next five minutes. "Lie down with your head near me and raise your feet." Sluggishly she responded. For the next few minutes I stroked her head and talked with her.

"What just happened? Has this ever happened before?"

"I have no idea. I took a drink and then I blacked out."

Eventually she sat up. "I have to go to the bathroom."

"I don't think you should. Just lie here for a while." I could tell she was barely in her body, still in a dissociative state.

"No, I have to go."

"Then hand me your cell phone." I'm not sure what I intended to do with it because I didn't know how to use a cell phone. She slid off the loveseat onto the floor and literally crawled into the bathroom. Eventually I heard the toilet flush and she walked back out and sat down.

Most handicap-accessible rooms with roll-in showers have only one king size bed so we slept together. When we went to bed that night, I kept my hand on her back all night to make sure she continued to breathe. Needless to say, I got very little sleep before my business meeting the next day!

I talked with my psychic friend, Cynthia, the next afternoon, recounting my experience.

"I felt absolutely helpless. I was watching someone quit breathing and possibly die right in front of me and I could do absolutely nothing."

"You're wrong. You brought her back," Cynthia reassured me.

"No, I didn't. I just called her name."

"Your energy brought her back. You saved her life."

She was adamant about helping me understand my role in the whole scenario.

"I wanted to get up and help her start breathing again. I couldn't. I was helpless."

"No, you weren't. It was your energy that brought her back. Never forget that."

To this day, the scene replays in my head. I wanted to help her physically and I couldn't. Perhaps because I'm unable to move physically, my mind has compensated by making me stronger mentally. I don't know. I'm just thankful that my first vacation in years didn't turn out to be a disaster. After a few hours of restless sleep, we met my business client for breakfast. Despite our frightening night, we never mentioned the ordeal to him. I summoned all of my professional façade an conducted business as usual.

Equipment Failure

Unfortunately, whenever you have to rely upon equipment for mobility, equipment failures are a given. Not too long ago I went to the grocery store and in the process of getting back into my van, my chair caught on a piece of plastic in the van. To understand this, you would have to own or have experience with a handicap converted van. The passenger seat is removed and replaced with a wheelchair lock down. Then a bolt is installed on the bottom of your wheelchair. When you go into the van, the bolt slides into the lockdown and keeps your wheelchair firmly in place for the ride.

On this particular day, the bolt caught on the plastic used to cover the carpeting in the van. I couldn't go forward and I certainly didn't want to try to back my way down the ramp. Many of my caregivers have a tendency to open the door on the opposite side of the van. Thank God it wasn't open that day.

My caregiver came behind me and slightly lifted the chair. You have to realize that the chair itself weighs 450 pounds even without my weight in it! As she lifted, I gunned the joystick full force. The chair jolted forward and slammed into the door on the opposite side of the van.

"Shit," I yelled. Both of my feet were bruised for days as a result of the crushing blow against the door.

Obviously, the interior door has a dent as a result of the mishap. All things considered, I was extremely fortunate that the opposite door had remained closed. Had it been open, I would've flown out of the opposite side of the van onto the curb and pavement below. I don't even want to imagine the amount of damage that would have caused my body. While my nervous system and feet took a jolt, I was not permanently injured. I try to always err on the side of caution but sometimes fate intervenes. On this occasion, I was just plain lucky.

On one other occasion a few years ago, I was not nearly so lucky. We were going to the store. It was the middle of winter here in northern Arizona with a cold rain pelting me as I left the house and raced to the van. As I was going up the ramp, the chair started to go off the ramp. I tried to correct it but it was too late.

Perhaps it was the combination of wet wheels on the chair and my desire to get into the warm van quickly that caused the ensuing disaster. In any case, I fell sideways off the edge of the ramp onto the hard garage floor still strapped to the chair. When my head hit the cement, it sounded like someone had taken a pumpkin, held it over his head and smashed it full force onto the floor. I laid there for a few seconds and wondered if I was dead. Surely someone could not survive that level of force.

Tina, my caregiver, had been getting into the van on the driver side when this happened. She came around the back of the van fully expecting to find me dead. Instead, I started to talk with her.

"We have to get me up."

"Oh my God, you are still alive. I can't believe it."

"The floor is damp and cold, can you tip me?"

The weight of the wheelchair with me strapped to it was simply too much for any one person to move. She ran inside the house to get the Hoyer lift to see if we could position me enough to use the Hoyer to lift me up. There was just no way that that was going to be possible.

"We have no choice," I said. "Call 911."

After running in the house to call 911, she came out and put a pillow under my head as we waited in the garage for the fire department to arrive. When they arrived, four guys lifted the chair and me into an upright position.

"Can you talk?" The leader of the EMT unit was questioning me.

"I can talk. I fell off the side of the ramp. I hit my head."

"Can you tell me what day it is?"

I answered his questions and then responded with the fact that I was alert times three. (Alert times three means that a person is alert to person, place and time.)

"My head slammed the cement very hard. And my shoulder hurts."

After feeling the lump on my head, one of the paramedics went into the house and grabbed an ice pack from the freezer while another paramedic asked questions about medications. They took my blood pressure. They took my glucose reading. After the trauma, my blood pressure was slightly elevated but not dangerously so.

"We want to transport you. What is the easiest way?"

"I don't want to be transported. I don't want to go to the ER."

"You really should be checked out. With the bump you've had on your head and your problems with your shoulder, you could have a concussion or worse. I would feel a lot better if we transported you."

Because I have had multiple sclerosis for over 30 years and have chosen not to become involved with Western medicine per se, I have always avoided or tried to avoid hospitals. I haven't taken any medication specifically for MS because I didn't want the side effects. I don't want to be a guinea pig. I don't want unnecessary tests. I don't want invasive procedures. I was concerned I would be exposed to all of that if I was taken to the hospital.

"I really think I'm okay. I know what to watch for with concussions. Can you tell me what software program you are using to record all of my vitals?"

The paramedic looked at me like I had just landed from outer space. "I sell medical software. I'm interested in how you are recording information. Can you show me?"

He turned his Toughbook tablet toward me and showed me the data input process. I was probably the only person who'd ever asked him to show their charting procedure. Because I own a software company called LifeSaver Group that features an online medical record, my curiosity was piqued. It is my intention that LifeSaverApp, our online medical record that is immediately available in the event of an emergency, will be interfaced with EMT units across the country in the near future.

The next day I called my primary care physician and told her what had happened. "What did they say at the ER?" she asked.

"I didn't go. They wanted to transport but I didn't want to go."

"You have got to be kidding me." I could almost see her shaking her head over the phone.

"No, I just didn't want to go. But I really need to have my shoulder checked out. It hurts a lot."

We scheduled an appointment for the next morning and after an examination and x-rays, it was determined I had broken my right clavicle – collarbone. No wonder it hurt so much. Because I had previously lost the use of my left arm after the accident in the kitchen where my neck had been so badly injured, I now lost the use of my one good arm. What hurt most was going up in straps in order to be transferred to the chair or to the bed or to the toilet. The only way I could handle the pain was to take a pain pill prior to the transfer.

My chiropractor helped during that time by adjusting the clavicle and using laser treatment on it to help it heal faster. Now it only bothers me on occasion when it is going to rain.

As for my head injury, again I was fortunate. I did not experience any brain bleed. I did, however, have nightmares about the sound of my head hitting the cement floor. To return to a sense of safety, my therapist talked me through the trauma using a technique called EMDR (Eye Movement Desensitization and Reprocessing). This psychotherapy treatment was originally designed to alleviate the distress associated with traumatic memories. Every once in a while I still have a flashback of that event as I'm going up the ramp into the van. For the most part, it's a constant reminder to be cautious.

Pilot Error or Mechanical Failure

Sometimes when quirky things happen, all you can do is laugh. One thing for certain: if you have mechanical equipment, something can and inevitably **will** go wrong. I have a power wheelchair that stands a person upright. While I would stand at home to stretch my legs, I had never used it when I went to the synagogue. One night I decided to stand during our standing prayer.

Since this was the first time I had ever stood in the synagogue, quite a few people turned around to look at me. The rabbi had a somewhat shocked look on her face. After the prayer ended, I remained standing. My standing power chair refused to sit down.

Without skipping a beat, the rabbi looked at me with a quizzical look and raised her eyebrows. I shrugged. Everyone turned around and looked at me. I just started laughing. What else could I do?

The rabbi's husband, Itzhak, got up and walked back to the row where I was still standing, red-faced of course.

"What can I do?" He started looking at my machine. When it comes to most equipment, he's quite mechanical. Standing power wheelchairs are controlled by computer chips and joysticks. When something goes wrong with them, it's not usually easy to fix.

"Nothing. Let me keep playing with it." I hit button after button trying to get it to release. Finally, it released and I sat back down. Needless to say, I didn't stand up again for the rest of the service!

The next day I called the manufacturer of the power chair and asked where the emergency release was.

"There is none," I was told.

"Let me speak to the owner, please." My call was transferred to the owner of the company.

"I was at synagogue over the weekend and decided to stand for prayer. My chair locked up and it wouldn't come back down. What do you do in a situation like that?"

"Call 911."

"You have got to be kidding me." I was astounded at his nonchalant response. "That is your solution? You haven't engineered any type of emergency release for this situation?"

"We've only had it happened a couple of times in our many years of business."

"That's no excuse. If it can happen to me, it can happen to other people." By this time, I was getting angry about his insensitivity. "What if your wife was in the chair and it happened to her? How would you feel about that? Would you want to call 911 and have fire department personnel carry her out of a public meeting?"

"Our company has an excellent track record. Unfortunately, you just experienced a fluke."

That was the official company response to my dilemma. When it came time to buy a new chair a couple of years ago, I remembered all too well their insensitivity. I purchased a new chair from a different company. As far as I was concerned, the scenario was definitely not pilot error; it was mechanical failure.

I have experienced instances of pilot error too. One night I was pulling up to the kitchen table in my chair. I accidentally ran into one of the chairs, splitting the vein in my leg wide open. We went up to the local ER for stitches. When the nurse came into the room, he started asking the typical questions.

"What are your medical conditions?" I started to answer him but instead asked my caregiver to grab my wallet. I handed him my LifeSaverApp medical ID card and suggested he follow the instructions on the card. He logged into our online website and came back with my two page emergency medical report.

"Is everything on this report current?"

"Yes, it is."

"Where did you get this? This is awesome. This answers every question I need to ask."

"It is my software product. I designed it for specifically this purpose. It consolidates the medical records and makes them immediately available in the event of emergency."

"If a person was unconscious, this could be a lifesaver. Why doesn't everybody have it?"

I laughed. "That's my intent. We'll be releasing it shortly and I want to get our local community involved first. I know it can save lives. And we have made it so inexpensive, I don't know how anybody could turn it down."

"Neither do I," he confirmed. "I am going to talk with the doctor about it."

As I am writing this book, we will be rolling out the product next week through social media. I am excited! It has taken years of programming and refinements to get it to the point where it can save lives and also serve as a missing person's report for conditions such as Alzheimer's where people wander away.

We know it could be the key to fixing the broken healthcare system in this country by providing immediate access to current medical information, avoiding unnecessary and duplicate tests while saving a person's life. If anyone from Shark Tank reading this book, please contact me!

You Need to Get Away

When you can walk, you don't really think about the things you take for granted on a daily basis. Everyone needs to get away occasionally including people who are disabled. If I want to travel or just go to a hotel in a different city for a couple of days, the experience becomes a major undertaking. Kirie and I decided to go to a cabin in Happy Jack, Arizona, for a couple of days in the middle of summer. We were assured that even though it was extremely hot in Sedona, the air would be cool in Happy Jack because it was at higher elevation and always cool.

When we arrived, the thermometer read 93°. The first obstacle presented itself as we tried to get through the door of the handicapped cabin. A lip my power chair couldn't traverse barred entry over the threshold. A bolt on the bottom of my power chair only allows about one inch clearance from the ground. The bolt is used as a locking device when I travel in the van, but unfortunately, it catches on many thresholds and doesn't allow entry into buildings. The maintenance man came and built a tiny ramp. First obstacle handled.

Once inside, more challenges presented themselves. The bathroom, while having a roll-in shower, was so small that the Hoyer lift couldn't be navigated to get to the toilet much less the shower. Because I cannot use my legs to transfer, everything has to be accessible using a portable lift. Much like my ceiling lifts, the Hoyer raises my body using a set of straps.

After everything was unloaded and put away in the cabin, I sat outside on the deck. The interior of the cabin was over 90°. A slight breeze cooled the deck a bit. After looking forward to getting away for a couple of days, I was now near tears. It all seemed so impossible.

"Do you want to go grab something to eat at that little diner?" Kirie asked as she emerged from the cabin. "Unless I'm mistaken, that's the only place to eat for miles."

"I think you're right. It's a little early for dinner but let's go ahead and grab something to eat."

When we arrived at the diner, we noticed only two or three cars in the parking lot. From the outside, it looked a little run down, but at least it was accessible. We went into the diner as Kirie held the door open for me. The menu was plastered against the back wall, above a counter. Small tables were scattered throughout with a couple of patrons making small talk. I figured they were probably local to the area. Compared to the outside, the inside of the diner was even more suffocating due to the heat of the kitchen.

"Oh my God, they don't have air conditioning."

"Obviously not," Kirie remarked as she lowered herself to the chair. Everything seemed more impossible by the minute. Once we decided what to order, Kirie walked to the front and placed the order.

"How about if we eat outside? It's cooler out there than in here."

"Totally agree. In fact, I think I'm going to go outside right now."

I left the restaurant and looked around the parking lot. The sun was beating down hard. The only shade was under a tree at the far end of the parking lot. When Kirie emerged with our food, I suggested we head toward the shade. Once we got to the edge of the parking lot, however, we could find no place to sit. We finally pulled the van into the shade and ate dinner with our lunch on our knees.

As I looked out the windshield, I saw a path leading up into the pines. It was blocked so a wheelchair couldn't get to it. At the end of the path was an outhouse. That was directly in front of our van. Looking to the side, a huge dumpster blocked most of the view. To find shade, we literally had to park in front of the shithouse alongside a dumpster. The food itself was presentable but the rest of the smells, not so much!

When we finished our meal, we went back to the cabin. I stayed outside rather than go into the hotbox.

Kirie came out of the cabin and pulled up a chair next to me. "What are you thinking?"

"I'm just so damn hot. It's a little bit better out here because there's a slight breeze."

"How are we possibly going to do this?"

I shook my head. "I don't know. I'm not even sure you can get me into the bed. And I don't know if it's even going to cool down tonight. Without air conditioning, I'm losing function fast."

"I know. I see that." We sat in silence for a few minutes, both lost in thought. Finally, I broached the topic I had been avoiding.

"I think we need to go home. I don't know how we can make this work."

"I was afraid you were going to say that. I know you are too hot. I don't know how I'm going to get you into bed."

"I don't know either. And I don't even want to go back into the cabin. I finally feel cooled down a little sitting out here."

After more discussion, Kirie packed up everything from the cabin and we returned to Sedona, hot, tired and defeated. It was just too hard to get away.

Nevertheless, we tried again. This time we went close by to a cabin up the canyon on 89A. It is only a few miles from our house in a beautiful setting next to the creek. Prior to checking in, we actually viewed the cabin for accessibility on the entryway. I knew the bathroom wasn't accessible but we were going to accommodate that inconvenience with a bedpan.

Packing everything in the van, we went up to the resort. After spending a quiet evening lounging by the fireplace and playing Rummikub, we decided to go to bed. The room had a king size bed, but no space on either side of the bed to maneuver the Hoyer lift. Getting me into the bed proved to be such a major accomplishment that the casual mood of the evening was ruined. The next day, I went back home, again defeated.

Now when people say to me "you need to get away for a few days," I smile wryly. It sounds nice in theory, but in reality, nothing is relaxing about it. Getting away is more work than staying home.

Taking the Simple Things for Granted

No book about disability would be complete without talking about the simple things in life "walkies" take for granted. Let's start with airline travel. Of course, everyone hates the check-in process necessitated by all of the security protocols nowadays. The last time I flew it went like this.

A security officer came over to me sitting in my wheelchair and said, "Can you please stand up and walk through the checkpoint?"

"No, I can't. I can't walk."

With a disgruntled look, he continued, "Can you at least stand up if I push you into the checkpoint?"

"No, really. I cannot walk. I cannot stand. I have absolutely no way to go into your checkpoint except by going through it in my chair."

An exasperated sigh followed. "Go over there," he said pointing to an area away from the line of people waiting to go through security. "I'll have to get a female officer to pat you down."

I left my fellow travelers and sat off to the side waiting for a female officer. It took at least 10 minutes before anyone came to frisk me. I'm not sure where I could have hid a weapon. In my bra? Oh no, I wasn't wearing one! In my underwear? Not hardly. In any case, imagine the loss of dignity when everyone is watching as you get patted down.

Once we arrived at the terminal, the check-in process began. Because I'm handicapped, I get to board first. Unfortunately, though, the boarding process is not easy. Instead of allowing handicapped people to remain in their own wheelchair, airline personnel transfer you from your wheelchair to a straight-backed chair. Because airlines are short of service staff now, they have to call to get people who can assist with the transfer. At first, a little short woman came up to me.

"I'll transfer you," she offered.

I just looked at her and laughed. Even though I was sitting down, I was practically eye level with her. In addition, I knew there was no way she could lift me. "You cannot possibly transfer me alone. My legs do not work. I can't stand. It takes a two-person transfer."

"I'm sure I can do it."

"Even if you were a big burly man, I wouldn't let you do it alone. I don't want you to hurt yourself and I certainly don't want to be dropped."

Reluctantly, she scurried away and looked for another person to help. I was holding up the boarding of the plane. She found a maintenance man to help. While he lifted underneath my arms, she lifted my legs and they got me into the straight-backed chair. Then they wheeled me to the airplane and took me on board.

When I got to my seat, I said, "This can't be right. I specifically told them I needed to be in a seat where the arm folded down."

"No, this is your seat. We can't change it now."

Between the two of them, they lifted me up and over the arm and into the seat. In the meantime, airport maintenance took my power chair, disassembled it and put it into baggage.

As an aside, I always cringe inwardly when I see them take my chair apart. During one trip to New York, they returned my chair from baggage but couldn't put it back together. They had somehow disconnected the electrical wiring so it didn't work at all. Luckily, my caregiver was handy mechanically so she fixed it.

On this trip, we flew to Phoenix. They brought the straight-back chair onto the plane and lifted me over the arm into the chair. Then they took me into the runway where my power chair was waiting. They lifted me out of the straight-backed chair into the wheelchair. Once I got to Sedona, I realized both of my breasts were bruised from the lifting and squeezing required to move me back and forth. Airlines could choose to have a locking mechanism that would allow handicapped people to use their own equipment and just be locked in place for the flight. Because it would require removing a seat from the aircraft to make it available for a handicapped person, not one single airline that has followed that suggestion. They don't want to lose any money by removing a seat! After all, occasionally a flight might exist without a disabled person on board. God forbid they should lose the money!

I quit traveling by air for another reason. If you can't walk, you can't get to the bathroom. I either had to be catheterized or wear a diaper. Within an hour of being catheterized, I get blood in my urine. It almost always results in a bladder infection. For that reason, I don't like being catheterized unless absolutely necessary.

One day during lunch in the middle of the seminar, I went up to my hotel room. I turned to my caregiver. "Do you think the people in the seminar have any idea I can't even dress myself or go to the bathroom without assistance?"

She shook her head. "I doubt it. You hide everything so well I doubt most people have a clue what you go through just to make a living."

When I first went to the synagogue, the rabbi told me about the wonderful handicapped bathroom in the synagogue. I have to agree. It is one of the largest and best equipped handicap bathrooms I have ever seen.

"I still can't use it. You have to be able to transfer to use the toilet. In my home, I have ceiling lifts that allow me to transfer to the bed, to the toilet, to the bathtub. Without them, I can't get where I need to be."

When I decide to go to services at the synagogue or out to a movie or to dinner, I always have to try to go to the bathroom before I leave. One of the problems with MS is the fact that you either have to go or you don't. There's nothing in between. I can't force myself to urinate even though I know my bladder is full. And then when I do have to go, it's immediate! I can't wait for five minutes or even one minute sometimes. That makes the decision to commit to an activity more difficult. My only other option is to wear a diaper.

When I first started to use a diaper or sanitary pad in case I needed to urinate before I got home, I was embarrassed. It is definitely a loss of dignity. Now, it has become a fact of life. Unless I am willing to give up socialization entirely, I need to use a diaper so I don't leak all over. Nothing can be worse than having urine run down your leg when you simply can't hold it! You can't hide that from anyone.

I used to try to quit drinking liquids by 5:00 p.m. at night so I didn't have to pee all night. Two years ago, I ended up in the hospital with acute interstitial nephritis – a nasty kidney infection that resulted in some amount of residual kidney damage. Rather than cut down on liquids at night, I sacrifice dignity and wear a diaper now. It just takes too long to get me out of bed in the middle of the night to go to the bathroom. It's not a matter of swinging your legs off the bed and running to the bathroom. It takes at least 10 minutes to get me hooked up in straps and even get a bedpan underneath me. It's definitely not sexy to wear a diaper but it is, however, a necessary evil.

The loss of dignity is incremental, occurring in small steps, eating away a little at a time.

The High Cost of Reality

One of my friends suggested I needed to include a section of the book talking about the physical costs of disability. Obviously, this book has dealt with the emotional costs and challenges. Most people don't want to know the monetary cost, but here is the truth.

Caregivers: If you need 24/7 caregivers and pay at least $12 per hour, that cost amounts to over $100,000 per year. Unless you were fortunate enough to have purchased long-term care insurance when you were healthy, this cost falls directly on you. Even with long-term care benefits, the coverage is limited and will run out.

Mobility products: Over the course of 30 plus years, I've probably purchased at least 12 different power chairs ranging from low-end scooters to high-end standing wheelchairs. A low-end scooter costs approximately $2,000. The last standing power chair I purchased was $38,000.

Ceiling lifts: So my caregivers don't have to lift me for any reason, I have installed ceiling lifts in the bedroom, the bathroom, the living room, and over the pool. Each ceiling lift costs $5000. You do the math! In addition, they have to be replaced periodically as the electronics or motors wear out. In all, I have probably purchased ten ceiling lifts. These lifts are imperative so my caregivers do not get hurt lifting me and I do not get dropped!

Handicap vans: Don't get me started on this one. I have had five handicapped-equipped vans. The first one was a full-size van with a lift. On snowy roads in Michigan, that van was an absolute danger. Even though it was heavy, it slid constantly. Since then, I've had four handicap-equipped minivans. I just priced a new one, swallowed hard, and said "No thank you." The list price is $65,000 for a Toyota Sienna with an in-floor lift. You can sometimes find used handicap vans with relatively low mileage. Of course, if you want to have an active life at all, you need to have decent transportation. A handicap-equipped van allows you to determine when and where you want to go.

Home modifications: Unless you are lucky enough to find the perfect home (and do they really exist), you must renovate to include entry ramps, wider doorways, lower countertops and removal of barriers. The cost of remodeling ranges between $500 and $10,000 depending on what you need.

Incidentals: I've listed the major equipment costs for mobility impairments. This doesn't include incidentals such as disposable and non-disposable bed pads, adult diapers, chair pads, adult wipes, etc. Believe it or not, I actually have a monthly subscription through Amazon for the ongoing monthly purchases.

Computers and software: To write this book, I used voice dictation software. Since I only have use of my right hand, it would have been an ungodly undertaking otherwise. The problem with voice dictation software is that it doesn't always understand you correctly so you have to make sure you error check thoroughly. I have been amazed and amused sometimes at the dictation errors.

I have been extremely blessed because my businesses have generated enough income to allow me to purchase the equipment and supplies I have needed. For that, I am exceptionally grateful.

I recently was asked what I missed most as a result of my mobility impairments. Here is a partial list to think of when you see someone in a chair:

I miss all of the activities that used to be so easy and enjoyable. I live in a city with over a thousand miles of awesome hiking trails. Our hiking trails are truly God's country. I can't hike any of them. I can't play golf on any of our beautiful golf courses. Any athletic activities I used to enjoy are now impossible.

Sometimes, it's nice to just climb in the car and take off. I miss the spontaneity of deciding on the spur of the moment to take a road trip. Deciding to go anywhere out of town takes a lot of preparation, and even then, it doesn't always turn out well.

One of the most difficult adjustments has been the necessity of always having someone in my home. I miss privacy. I have caregivers here 24/7. Too often, they listen to private conversations, comment on my choices in life, and attempt to force their beliefs into my personal space. One caregiver had the audacity to suggest that my MS was God's punishment for being a lesbian. I stress boundaries in every caregiver interview, but find too many people simply do not have a clue!

People who can walk and move their bodies with ease don't appreciate the gift of mobility. I miss many of the things people take for granted - like the ability to give someone a full body hug, the ability to stand up and leave if people around me are being obnoxious, the ability to do the simple things in life like bathe, dress, and even roll over in bed.

I experience unavoidable "time sucks" that can be inconvenient and downright disturbing. I used to take five-minute showers. Now I have to take baths which I figure has added an additional 20 minutes every day or 219,000 minutes so far in my lifetime. That's the equivalent of 3,650 hours, or 152 twenty-four hour days. Does that put it in perspective?

Trying not to laugh or drink when I go out. I miss being able to go to a restaurant or movie without worrying about whether or not I will have to go to the bathroom in the middle of it because I know even a handicap bathroom is inaccessible for me. For that reason, I avoid drinking beverages when I go to the restaurant or to a show. Sometimes, I even hesitate to laugh… and certainly sneeze… because a wet disaster lurks!

As people age, they eventually have to give up driving. I gave up driving over 20 years ago because I no longer felt it was safe, not only for me but for the other drivers on the road. When you use hand controls, you push away from you for the brake and push down for acceleration. Because my body goes into spasm when I get tired or hot, I no longer felt it was safe to drive. I cannot control the spasms. At first, it was just my legs. Now my arms go into spasm, my back, and even my chest muscles. I didn't want to use the car in front of me to stop when my body would go into total spasm! I once watched a gentleman pull into the parking lot at a physical therapy practice. He used the pylon to stop his car. When he got out of the car to go into the building for physical therapy, I could see why. He could barely walk. He had no business driving a car.

I've heard some organizations and classes attempt to sensitize people to the issues faced by individuals in wheelchairs. For 24 hours, class members have to navigate the world from a wheelchair. They have to attempt to go to the bathroom, open doors, go about their daily business from the perspective of a wheelchair user. They encounter first-hand the obstacles like lack of curb cuts, people parking in handicapped spots, thresholds too high to allow entrance, and the many daily challenges. I totally understand and appreciate the fact that attempts are being made to sensitize people to the issues from an educational perspective.

I have only one thing to add: after twenty-four hours, their sensitization stint is over. Imagine not being able to get up and walk away from the wheelchair. That is the reality many of us face.

Tongue-In-Cheek

My editor suggested I needed to include the positive things I have gained from being in a chair. So here's a list:

Standup comedian – I have always wanted to be a standup comedian. Now I need to settle for being a sit down comic.

Driving Miss Daisy – Because I can't drive myself, I get to play *Driving Miss Daisy* every time I go somewhere. Considering the way some people drive and I can't be a backseat driver, my attitude sometimes matches Miss Daisy!

Saving on essentials – Since I don't walk, I don't wear out shoes quickly. And, because I'm always sitting, I choose not to wear underwear. It takes too long to get the underwear off when I have to go to the bathroom quickly. See how much money I'm saving! What an incentive to be permanently in a chair.

Ready-made roadkill – If someone upsets me or makes me angry, my 450-pound chair can be used as an instrument of destruction/torture. Of course, you have to make sure you're not accidentally making roadkill of a friend.

Standing room only – When the venue is standing room only (SRO), I don't have to worry about finding a seat!

Getting out of chores – I don't have to take out the garbage because I can't carry it while I work the joystick on my chair. I don't have to load the dishwasher because I can't bend over that far. I don't have to cook because I can't reach the stove. Being in a chair gives me a built-in excuse for getting out of chores. I don't have to pretend I want to do it but I'm just lazy.

Lightning strike – In the event of a lightning strike, I am automatically grounded by my rubber tires. I have the perfect excuse for standing out (sitting out) in a thunderstorm.

Scripts for a new TV serial - With all of the drama of daily life with caregivers, I could write enough scripts for a 10-year run of Caregiver Hell! It would definitely be an alternate reality show.

Knowing more than doctors – During the beginning stages of MS, one of the symptoms was hyperactive reflexes. As I was being examined by a young intern, he was standing directly in front of me as he proceeded to test my knee-jerk reflex. I gently pointed out to him that he might want to step to the side if he ever wanted to have children!

Knee replacements – Many people my age have worn out their knees and are keeping the medical establishment in business through knee replacements. One big advantage of not walking is the fact that you don't have to replace your knees.

You can't grab it – because I'm sitting on my bottom, you can't grab my… LOL

What is the Lesson?
When I was first facing the effects of MS, I asked the typical question, "Why me, God?"

The only answer I ever received was "why not?" Indeed, why not? As much as we like to believe we're in control of our lives, our world can spiral out of control in a split second. I'm not sure how people without a belief in a higher power would handle a chronic illness or disability. I don't think I could without my belief – it sustains me when everything else feels bleak.

New Age philosophy suggests we experience many lifetimes and in the interim between lifetimes, we decide on the lessons we want to learn in the next lifetime. While this philosophy is a convenient explanation, I can't help but wonder who would choose physical disability as a lesson. Was I really that naive?

An alternate philosophy is the thought that we choose difficult lessons to elevate ourselves more quickly. Okay, nice thought, but really? I think I would rather come back a few more times than try to learn it all at once. Sometimes I can't help but think about the trails I haven't been able to hike, the golf courses I haven't been able to play, the camping trips I haven't been able to take, or the places I've always wanted to visit like Switzerland, Israel, and Hawaii. So many things are totally out of reach, impossible. I need to return to this planet at least one more time to experience the things I haven't been able to experience in this lifetime.

For anyone dealing with a chronic illness such as multiple sclerosis, cancer, diabetes, kidney disease, you name it, we all have one thing in common. If your disease is in remission, there is a daily fear that it will recur. You can push away the fear, but it's never 100% gone. If your disease like MS, has a tendency to get worse over time, you wonder every time you get sick – do I have the flu or is my MS getting worse? Sometimes it's hard to distinguish between a common cold and the worsening of a chronic disease.

Some things we know for sure about MS. Most people find their symptoms get worse when they have an infection in any part of the body, when they fall, when they get too hot since most people with MS are heat sensitive and when they are under stress. It is almost impossible to avoid all of these triggers. Many of these same triggers are present for other chronic disease processes.

Dealing with caregivers on a daily basis adds to the stress level. Every person comes with their own emotional baggage and, unfortunately, the bags are not carry-ons that can be stowed in compartments. In addition, caregivers also bring their physical ailments. If they have a cold, you are exposed to a cold. If they have flu, you are exposed to the flu. Because young children carry so many germs, most of the time I prefer to hire older people. The germs carried by young children are virulent and extremely hard to get rid of! Once they latch on to you, they are like a parasite – you can't get rid of them.

If I were to find a lesson in all of this, it's the ability to appreciate the small things in life. Going out to a movie or dinner with a friend. Sitting in the park surrounded by nature. Lounging next to Oak Creek as it trickles its way down the mountain.

One day as I was praying at my medicine wheel, I asked the universe for peace. When I woke up one day realizing that the universe had recognized and fulfilled my intention, I observed an interesting correlation. Along with peace comes the presence of joy. No one can take away your peace or your joy. You can choose to give it away but no one can forcibly take it from you. Peace and joy are yours for the asking.

Why Did I Choose Judaism?

Because my rabbi is also my friend and a voracious reader, I shared the first draft of my book with her. She called me immediately after finishing the book. "First of all, you absolutely need to get this published. You have insight that will be helpful for so many people. This book isn't just for you."

While writing this book has been somewhat of a catharsis, it has also put issues in my face. Nevertheless, I responded, "That's my intention. I wanted to have you read it first and make sure I didn't misrepresent Judaism in any way."

We talked for a couple of minutes about the various concepts in the book. Then she asked, "Why did you choose Judaism? With all of your experiences including channeling and an astral trip and Native American ritual, why choose Judaism? What was there about it that appealed to you?"

Her question took me aback. Here was my rabbi questioning my decision to become a Jew! I realized when I chose Judaism I added another target on my back. I was already a lesbian and disabled. Both of those facets of my life put a target on my back. Becoming a Jew by choice added yet another target. As I write this book, the political climate and conservative agenda have intensified all of my targets. I have the perfect trifecta without a winning ticket! So why did I become a Jew by choice?

"Being raised Christian, I couldn't buy into some of the dogma. For example, I could not under any circumstances accept the concept of original sin. How can a newborn baby be a sinner? I just couldn't accept that."

In my mind, I could see her nodding her head in agreement. "You are absolutely right. We believe the soul of a baby is pure. When it gets shmutzed up, we are given the tools to 'clean it up' and get back to our original pure soul each morning with the morning blessings, each week on Shabbat, each month with the new moon, and certainly during the introspective preparation for the High Holy Days when we take responsibility for any wrongdoings."

"Exactly. And I couldn't just swallow the concept of original sin. I also don't like some of the misinterpretations of the Bible. I like the fact that Judaism encourages people to disagree. Rabbis even take opposing views of the same line of Scripture. For example, today in Torah study when we talked about Moses and the burning bush."

"Yeah, that was an animated discussion wasn't it?"

"Definitely! I sat and listened as people threw ideas back and forth across the table. It was fascinating the number of different interpretations of the burning bush."

Rabbi Alicia agreed. "It was. Everyone had something to contribute. Why did Moses see the burning bush and no one else did? How did the bush burn without being consumed? Lots of questions with no definitive answer. Why did Moses have to turn to see it? Surely a burning bush would've been obvious, literally in your face."

"And that's what I like. I like the challenge of it. And I like the fact there is no one right answer. One of the interpretations really struck home. What if Moses was the only one who saw the burning bush because it was only in his head?"

Again, I saw the Rabbi nodded in agreement in my mind. "Yeah, that is an interesting interpretation."

"I also like the fact that you, the rabbi, speak and read Hebrew fluently. Going back to the original language changes the interpretation of how we understand the Hebrew Bible. It made me ask about words from later biblical texts. Many mis-translations have found their way into the New Testament that I read as a child such as the description of Mary as a virgin when, in the original Hebrew, really referred to a young woman. How far off is that? Obviously, it was changed drastically during the translation from Hebrew/Aramaic to Greek to English."

She asked me, "Have you considered adding anything to your book about your decision to become Jewish?"

"I might add a chapter," I responded. "And maybe at a later date, I will write another book comparing my thoughts on Christianity and Judaism. It wouldn't be an intellectual exercise. It would definitely be a more emotional response."

Since our discussion a few days ago, I have given such a book more thought. At some point, I may decide to write that book. I certainly have explored spirituality from many different aspects prior to finding my home in Judaism. They say home is where the heart is. I found my home in Judaism. And now I will explain my Hebrew name.

What is in a Name?

When a baby's birth is imminent, most parents spend time choosing a name. In my case, I am named after my mother. My first name is her middle name. My middle name, Kay, was chosen because Kay was a nurse friend of my mother's.

When you convert to Judaism, you have the opportunity to choose your Hebrew name. As my beit din* approached, I was talking with Rabbi Alicia about the ceremony.

"You need to choose your Hebrew name," she reminded me.

"I know."

"Your name, Marilyn, is close to Miriam, Moses' sister. She was a prophetess. She helped lead our people out of Egypt. It's a powerful name. That would be a good name for you."

I nodded my head in agreement. "She was certainly instrumental in history. I have no doubt about that."

I have the utmost respect for Rabbi Alicia. Part of me wanted to allow her to choose my name, but I had been doing research for my name. Earlier in my life, people kept giving me buffaloes. Buffalo statues, buffalo pictures, buffalo sayings. Everywhere I looked, I had buffaloes. Eventually, my house looked like a herd of buffalo. Thank God, it wasn't accompanied by buffalo chips. For those who don't know, buffalo chips are dry dung used as fuel!

As I got into Native American ritual, I looked up the meaning of buffalo as a totem. Once I realized the meaning of buffalo, it started to make sense. Buffalo stands for abundance and prayer. To the Native American, buffalo is sacred. When a buffalo life was taken, it provided food, shelter, and clothing. I wanted my Hebrew name to reflect my belief in abundance.

Don't you love Google? What did we do prior to the Internet? I typed "abundance in Hebrew" and found that "shefa" means abundance in Hebrew. I knew immediately that shefa was part of my name. The second part of my name "lev" means heart. My entire Hebrew name is Shefa Lev bat Avraham v'Sarah.

I somewhat hesitantly told Rabbi Alicia the name I had picked for myself. "I really like Shefa Lev," I offered. "I have been doing research to find a name that resonates with me. I like Miriam but it doesn't resonate with me."

Instead of showing disappointment in my choice, the rabbi clapped enthusiastically. "That is so perfect! The abundance of love flowing through you from the Divine above and outward from your heart. I love that name for you." In her theatrical way, her hand reached toward the heaven as she acted out my name.

I breathed a sigh of relief.

"You have chosen a great name."

What's in a name? Our identity. In my case, I had the opportunity to choose how I wanted to be identified in my chosen religion.

My friend Anita interpreted my name recently in Torah study. The interpretation is as follows: abundant love, light, and wisdom flow through her from the depths of her heart and the heavenly heights above, spreading her influence of *tikkun olam*** throughout the world.

I chose the name. It is my challenge and responsibility to live up to it. Whew!

*A beit din is a panel of three rabbis who question a perspective Jew-by-choice to determine if the person has taken adequate preparation to become a Jew.

** *Tikkun olam* means to repair the world, to perform activities that improve the world bringing it into a more harmonious state. It is the responsibility and privilege of every Jew to perform *Tikkun olam*.

Prayer for Healing

One of my favorite parts of a Shabbat service is the congregational prayer for healing. Debbie Friedman put the prayer to music and it's used in synagogues throughout the world.

In our synagogue, prior to singing Mi Shebeirach, the rabbi passes her hand through the congregation as we call out names of people we want to include for healing prayers. Then the entire congregation sings the song made famous by Debbie.

Mi shebeirach avoteinu
M'kor hab'racha l'imoteinu
May the source of strength,
Who blessed the ones before us,
Help us find the courage to make our lives a blessing,
and let us say, Amen.

Mi shebeirach imoteinu
M'kor habrachah l'avoteinu
Bless those in need of healing with r'fuah sh'leimah,
The renewal of body, the renewal of spirit,
And let us say, Amen.

If you would like to hear Mi Shebeirach being sung, go to YouTube.com and type Debbie Friedmman with the title of the song.

The many different views on healing are endless. From my perspective, it would take a true miracle for me to ever walk again. Honestly, I can't imagine that happening. From my perspective, I can't imagine what it would feel like to regain sensory perception in my arms and legs. I can't imagine that happening either. Of course, neither would I turn it down!

For me, healing has taken the form of acceptance. Realizing my life will always have limitations has been a journey. While many people experience failing health as they age, it's rare to experience disability during the prime years of your life unless you've had a devastating accident.

Whatever your challenge in life, it is my prayer something in this book helps you face it head on with the strength of spirit.

A famous quote from our Talmudic sage Rabbi Tarfon: It is not your responsibility to finish the work, but neither are you free to desist from starting it. (*Pirkei Avot*) It was my responsibility to write this book. The response to the book is in God's hands.

Tribute to Debbie Friedman

While Debbie has moved on to a "place that we do not know," her spirit lives on in the inspirational music she left to all of us.

She continues to be a blessing...

If you want to know more about Debbie Friedman, her life and the impact on Jewish liturgy, look up her information on YouTube.

Her website is: http://www.debbiefriedman.com

About the Author

Marilyn Gard can be reached via the following email or website addresses.

Email: marilyn@clinicpro.com

Websites:

LifeSaverGroup: www.lifesavergroup.com

LifeSaverApp: www.lifesaverapp.com

911SafeChild: www.911safechild.com

911Assets: www.911assets.com

ClinicPro software: www.clinicpro.com

Personal website: www.marilynkgard.com

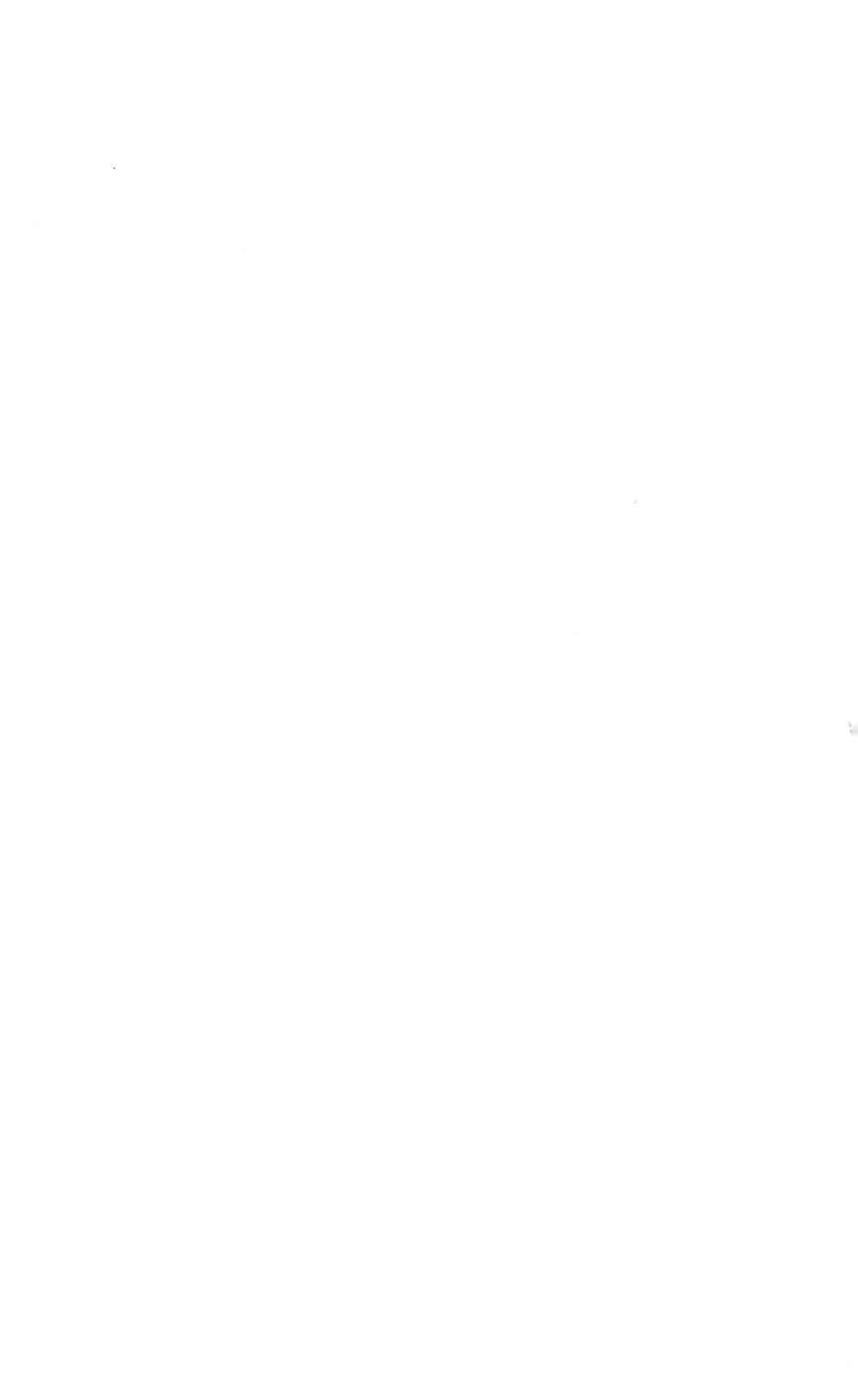

Made in the USA
Columbia, SC
13 October 2023